Aromatherapy and Massage

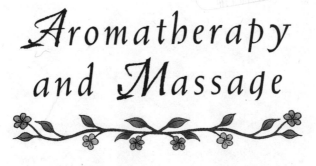

FOR MOTHER AND BABY

Aromatherapy and Massage

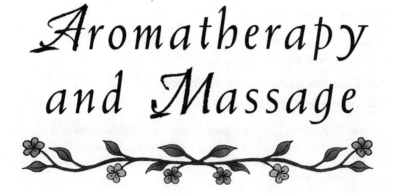

FOR MOTHER AND BABY

ALLISON ENGLAND

Healing Arts Press
Rochester, Vermont

Healing Arts Press
One Park Street
Rochester, Vermont 05767
www.InnerTraditions.com

Healing Arts Press is a division of Inner Traditions International

*Note to the reader: This book is intended as an informational guide. The remedies,
approaches, and techniques described herein are meant to supplement, and not to be a
substitute for, professional medical care or treatment. They should not be used to treat
a serious ailment without prior consultation with a qualified health care professional.*

Library of Congress Cataloging-in-Publication Data

England, Allison.
  Aromatherapy and massage for mother and baby / Allison England.
    p. cm.   6506375
  Rev. and expanded edition of Aromatherapy for mother and baby.
  Includes bibliographical references and index.
  ISBN 0-89281-898-0
    1. Aromatherapy. 2. Pregnant women—Health and hygiene. 3. Infants—Health
and hygiene. I. England, Allison. Aromatherapy for mother and baby. II. Title.

RG525 .E538 2000
615'.321—dc21
                                                          99-089913

Printed and bound in the United States

10 9 8 7 6 5 4 3 2 1

This book was typeset in Bembo with Nuptial Script as the display typeface

615.321
Eng

To my children

Contents

Acknowledgments

First and foremost I would like to thank Shealgh Doyle for her support and encouragement—without her this book would never have gotten onto paper.

My grateful thanks for their help and time go to midwife Ailsa Dale, for her advice and for taking the time to write a foreword showing such enthusiasm for aromatherapy; Lola Borg for sorting out and editing the manuscript while having a baby (Francis) and moving; and my clients, without whom there would have been no knowledge gained.

Special thanks and love go to my husband, Michael, for his loyal encouragement; and my children, Nick, Charlotte, Sophie, Ben, and William, for the summer vacation over all too quickly, the goodies they kept me going with, and all the many, many meals they shopped, cooked, and washed up for without too much of a grumble!

Foreword

Aromatherapy is escalating in popularity and what a good thing that is, since essential oils are, in my opinion, safe, nontoxic, and extremely pleasant to use.

I am a midwife at a district general hospital that has 2,500 deliveries annually. I mainly work on a ward for prenatal and postnatal women where essential oils are now available. In 1986 some of my colleagues introduced me to aromatherapy. They already used oils personally and suggested that I start using them in our holistic approach to individualized care. One of the great things about aromatherapy is watching my friends become converted. My husband—the greatest skeptic of all—now uses oils in his bath every Saturday to ease his rugby-injured muscles.

Following a daylong workshop by an aromatherapist, I confidently introduced lavender oil into the ward environment in 1987. A year later, a quality assurance survey showed that 84 percent of the patients who had used essential oils had found them useful. Most women find relief and comfort from a long warm bath containing lavender oil. It eases the pain of early labor; it cleanses and seems to help heal perineal wounds following childbirth. Lavender oil also balances moods in that most emotionally unstable of times.

We now make regular use of five different essential oils, giving individual tuition to new midwives who want to help patients use them. They are told how many drops to use and the dangers of side effects if they are used inappropriately. Once advised about the oils, patients have access to them and may self-administer them in bathwater, in massage, or as compresses or inhalations.

Until recently the value of aromatherapy was purely anecdotal. Now several people have started researching the use of essential oils, so in the future the medical profession will have to accept the claims made for them and will, I hope, promote this lovely alternative.

Ailsa Dale
Midwife, Hinchingbrooke Hospital
Huntingdon, England

Introduction

As a practicing aromatherapist, I have enjoyed working with people of all ages and types. Over the last few years, however, I have begun to take a particular interest in the health of women during and after pregnancy, probably fueled by my own experiences as a mother of five children. Pregnancy is a special time in a woman's life, and I feel she deserves to be taken care of while she is taking care of her baby.

I have seen the health of many pregnant women improve during a course of aromatherapy treatments, just as I've witnessed other women who are in good health remain in top form. Patients also look to me for reassurance, and I think that like a mother, an aromatherapist often has to be counselor, dietitian, nurse, and friend who is good at listening, all rolled into one.

This book was based on the many questions I have been asked by mothers-to-be and new mothers with whom I've shared my love of essential oils. It was conceived because I felt that these particular women needed to fully understand how to use these powerful aromatic oils to their very best advantage—and there are indeed many advantages.

But wonderful as they are, essential oils should be treated with respect. Just because they are a natural product from the plant world does not mean they can be used without thought and care. I'm sure you are familiar with what I call the grandmother touch—the philosophy that an extra spoonful would do you a world of good. Although well intentioned, this philosophy should never be applied when using essential oils, where less often means more. Like all things in life, our bodies need balance. We thrive on vitamins and minerals, for example, and they are naturally found in our bodies. All is well when the correct amount is taken; but too much of a good thing can provoke a negative reaction. For this reason, essential oils are excellent for use by pregnant women and the very young, but they need to be chosen and used with great care.

Aromatherapy has quite rightly gained tremendous popularity in recent years. The enthusiastic flair with which journalists have written about it in magazines has encouraged many readers to try these exotic oils. However, few people, even those keenly interested in complementary therapies, fully understand its origins and applications. I will describe aromatherapy in this book, particularly how it can help you through pregnancy and early motherhood.

You have so much to look forward to as a prospective mother (or father). Aromatherapy can play a small part in making the experience more fulfilling.

1

The Benefits of Aromatherapy in Pregnancy

I see many mothers-to-be in my aromatherapy practice, and each approaches her pregnancy differently. Some are excited and positive in their outlooks, they feel well, and they strive to be in the very best of health. Others are apprehensive—they feel they are entering unknown territory and worry about every aspect of pregnancy and birth, from losing their figure to how they will cope with the new baby. Many worry that their relationship with their partner will change. Some women are not in peak condition and find that the myriad discomforts of pregnancy—particularly in the last few months—leave them physically or emotionally drained, especially if they already have a family to care for.

New mothers, of course, have their own problems. They may be tired from feeding or from the constant activity that comes with a new baby, and perhaps they must cope with the aftereffects of a cesarean birth or an episiotomy.

The wonderful thing about aromatherapy is that it has something to offer all these women. Aromatherapy is an entirely individual treatment aimed at making each mother feel her very best. It can be used to help prevent or cope with problems that may arise in pregnancy or early motherhood. Mothers can turn to aromatherapy for very different reasons, and in each case it will be appropriate and beneficial. It can provide nurturing, nourishing treatment that will enhance well-being and self-awareness, and it can help relieve minor ailments.

WHERE AROMATHERAPY HELPS MOST

Some of the most important ways in which aromatherapy can help you enjoy your pregnancy and your new baby are listed below.

- It can help you deal with stress.

- It will aid relaxation, help develop a more positive outlook, and, therefore, help with the birth. A happy, relaxed mother is one who is more likely to cope well with labor and to relax and bond with her baby afterward.

- It can help with tiredness, aches, and pains, and it can provide relief from all kinds of minor ailments that result during pregnancy. It can back up and complement what is learned at relaxation and prenatal classes. Women who have had aromatherapy are more likely to benefit from the relaxation techniques they learn.

- It can help prevent stretch marks by keeping the skin well nourished, and it can aid in helping the mother feel good about herself during her pregnancy.

- Mothers-to-be who experience the benefits of aromatherapy are more likely to be in touch with their bodies and their pregnancies, which benefits both mother and baby.

- The caring touch of a massage, either from a qualified aromatherapist or from a partner, is highly therapeutic. A woman who can appreciate the touch and care she receives while being massaged is more likely to bond well with her baby using her own tactile sense.

After an aromatherapy massage, a mother-to-be will often report a feeling of extreme peace and well-being. Her face may take on a look of tranquility. The massage can also help relieve the tensions in her life. Naturally, aromatherapy cannot remove the day-to-day problems that life throws at us, but someone who is relaxed can deal with them all the better. The best way to receive an aromatherapy massage during pregnancy is from a qualified practitioner (see appendix 1 to find one in your area), but having a massage from your partner at home is beneficial as well.

SUCCESS STORIES

To give you a clearer idea of the benefits of aromatherapy in pregnancy, I have included accounts of patients I have treated, either while pregnant or postpartum, in my aromatherapy practice.

CAMILLA

Camilla came to see me when she was four months pregnant with her fourth child. She was tense and tired, said she wasn't sleeping well, and had been told aromatherapy might help. At first her answers to my general questions about her health were brusque; eventually she broke down into sobs.

She had recently returned to full-time teaching after what she described as "years at home" with her children who were now thirteen, eleven, and six years old. She had been delighted with her job but knew it would be hard to manage with a family. She had believed they could muddle through, however. Suddenly she felt everything had gone wrong. Unlike her other pregnancies, the current one was taking its toll on her. She was snappy and on edge; she felt overwhelmed and couldn't cope with the exhausting demands of working all day, running a home, and looking after her family. She was worried about how she would cope with the new baby, even with the help of a babysitter. She didn't want to resign from her job because she felt she might not get another chance like it again; her husband was building up a new business after being laid off and they needed the extra money.

Camilla had always been a "manager" and never liked to ask for help, but she agreed to talk to her husband and explain to him how tired she was and to lighten her load by getting friends to help out occasionally with her after-school commitments, such as taking her daughter to ballet classes. She agreed to tell her doctor that she was feeling low, but I suggested that for the moment we should concentrate on making her feel better within herself so that she could relax and sleep more soundly. Aromatherapy cannot wave a magic wand over problems, but I believed that if she felt less tired and was in a more positive frame of mind, she would be in a better position to find some solutions to her problems.

Camilla loved the smell of the neroli oil I used to massage her, saying that the smell alone made her feel more cheerful. Although she was tense when I began her first massage, she was far more relaxed by the time I had finished. She provisionally booked another appointment with me for the following week.

The very next day I received a phone call from Camilla. She had slept for the first time in weeks and asked if I could see her in three days instead of in a week. She continued to come twice weekly for three weeks and then weekly for the rest of her pregnancy. She called it her "hour of bliss."

To back up Camilla's treatment, I mixed a relaxing bath oil of ylang-ylang, neroli, and lavender. Her husband also used the bath oil and reported that it helped him unwind at night and sleep well. I also made up a body oil with mandarin and lavender to ease her aching back, legs, and feet.

Camilla remained physically healthy for the remainder of her pregnancy. The occasional leg ache was soothed by a foot massage given by her husband or eldest son (albeit for a bit of extra pocket money). She still had her job and family to juggle, but because she was feeling better and coping well, she began to look forward to the birth. She became much more relaxed about delegating chores to the rest of the family and putting her feet up in the evenings.

After a very short labor, during which her sister-in-law (who was Camilla's chosen birth partner) massaged her with lavender oil, Camilla gave birth to a beautiful baby girl.

JANE

Jane was a physiotherapist who was familiar with aromatherapy. She sometimes used essential oils at the end of her patients' treatments to ease their aches and pains. Her patients, she said, enjoyed the "hands-on approach" of massage, especially because so many physiotherapy treatments seemed to be performed by machines. She had also been impressed by the pain-relieving qualities of the essential oils she had used on her patients. Now that she was pregnant, Jane wanted to receive some tender loving care instead of giving it.

This was Jane's first pregnancy, and she was feeling fit and well. During her initial consultation, I asked about the essential oils she used on her patients, particularly because the sort of ligament and joint conditions she worked with called for strong oils such as marjoram, juniper, and rosemary, none of which should be used during pregnancy. She assured me that as soon as she knew she was pregnant she had switched to gentler oils—lavender, chamomile, and sometimes sandalwood—and always in a low dilution.

Jane intended to keep on working as long as possible. She remained well throughout her pregnancy and really relaxed during her aromamassage each week. I used tangerine oil in a base of avocado and almond oil for her massage and mixed up a bottle for her to use at home. This oil helped to keep her skin supple to prevent stretch marks. She used this oil at night, but because she had to be out of the house quickly in the mornings and didn't have time to let it "sink in" before getting dressed, I also made a creamy, nonsticky tangerine gel, which she could apply liberally before dressing.

Toward the end of her pregnancy, Jane found, like many women on their feet all day, that her legs ached. I made her a gel with lavender and lemon—a wonderfully cooling recipe that drains the throb from aching legs and feet.

Jane had known early in her pregnancy that her baby was to be born by cesarean section. She now has a little boy who regularly enjoys an aroma baby massage from his mother.

JENNY

I never met Jenny personally, but shortly before her due date she contacted me with a very definite list of requirements. She wanted a relaxing bath oil for labor (and also one for her husband!), a labor massage oil with jasmine and lavender, and a soothing bath oil for after the birth. Her friend, she explained, had used aromatherapy during her pregnancy and recommended it.

I duly sent off a package and a month later received a very sweet, newsy letter. She had had twin boys and had been determined to have a drug-free birth. She had found the lavender and ylang-ylang bath oil I sent soothing and relaxing; under the watchful eye of the midwife, she had been allowed to stay in the bath for longer than she'd expected during the first stage of her labor. In fact, she said, the other midwives kept popping in to find out what the wonderful smell was. The jasmine and lavender massage oil had worked well for the second stage of her labor, and she hadn't needed any extra pain relief, much to the surprise of the nurses. She had been disappointed, though, that monitors had been attached to her abdomen at the end of the first stage and throughout the rest of the delivery to check the babies' heartbeats. The first twin was born quickly with good, strong contractions. With the second, however, she had to have her legs in stirrups. The baby was positioned awkwardly and there was a chance that forceps would be needed. Luckily, they weren't, and although she didn't have quite the "stand-and-deliver" type of birth she had planned, she was very happy to have given birth without drugs. She was overjoyed to be the proud mother of two beautiful boys.

Jenny received a few stitches but used the lavender and cypress bath oil I had sent. The nursing staff was surprised at how quickly she had healed. As for the bath oil for her husband: Yes, she reported, he had had some relaxing nights' sleep before the birth, so he was fit and ready when the twins went home.

MARY

I was initially contacted by Mary's mother-in-law, who was staying with her for two weeks while Mary's husband was on a business trip abroad. Mary was four weeks postdelivery. Jamie's birth had been long and difficult, and Mary just hadn't picked up afterward. She was tired and run down from coping with a new baby who wouldn't settle down in the evenings and a three-year-old daughter who constantly wanted her attention and who wouldn't go to bed at night. Mary's mother-in-law, who believed that bedtime was bedtime no matter what, felt that Mary was being far too liberal with her daughter. There was a lot of tension in the family.

Mary came to see me looking tired and washed out, with shadows under her eyes, dry skin, and limp hair. She said she felt utterly seedy and joked that her husband would probably take one look at her and jump back on the nearest plane.

Mary had breast-fed for the first two weeks after the birth but was supplementing with bottles because she was so tired and because Jamie cried so much she felt she wasn't satisfying him. She would have preferred just to breast-feed. We talked a little about life at home. She had been upset that her husband had had to go away on business, and even though she understood that it was necessary and that he had already delayed work to be at the birth, she felt she needed his support. Having his mother visit was a strain. She was very kind and she meant well, but she had a much more rigid way of doing things, whereas Mary preferred to take each day as it came. Mary admitted that hers might not always be the best approach, and she believed that Alex, her daughter, was acting up because of it.

I gave Mary a massage with geranium—a good, balancing pick-me-up oil—in a base of peach nut kernel oil. The base was good for her dry skin, but I used it mostly because she liked the sound of it. For the dry skin on her face, I used rose oil in jojoba, and she took a bottle of it home with her to use at night. I suggested a soothing bath each night with essential oils of lavender and bergamot to help her relax. I also suggested that she drink fennel tea to help increase her milk supply and take a rest during the day when the baby was sleeping, letting her mother-in-law amuse Alex in the afternoons instead of trying to do it herself. Mary had been keeping Alex with her all day because she was worried her daughter might feel jealous of the baby, but she admitted that even a small child can appreciate when her mother needs a little time alone. A loving grandmother was just the person to take over on those occasions.

With the help of a doll I keep especially for demonstration purposes, I showed Mary how to give a baby massage that would help her baby sleep if he had colicky pain. She agreed to try it after his morning bath to see if he liked it, so I made up a chamomile massage oil for him.

When Mary arrived the following week, she looked much better. Jamie had been a little suspicious of the first massage, but subsequent ones had done the trick and he was sleeping most evenings. He was more relaxed and so was Mary. Her mother-in-law had taken Alex out most afternoons while Mary took a nap, and Mary found that she was more relaxed in the evenings. Mary had stopped bottle-feeding Jamie and was breast-feeding frequently.

2

Aromatherapy and Essential Oils Explained

WHAT IS AROMATHERAPY?

The word *aromatherapy* means "treatment using scent," and that's exactly what it is. Aromatherapy is a therapeutic and complementary treatment that reaches the very core of our senses through touch and smell, using the scents from aromatic oils to heal and uplift the body and spirit and make us feel mentally and physically healthier.

Contrary to popular belief, aromatherapy is not just massage with scented oils. Aromatherapists do use massage as an important and very valuable part of many treatments, but they also use oils in other ways, too—for aromatic baths and in creams, lotions, compresses, and vaporizers.

ESSENTIAL OILS

Essential oils are highly concentrated and potent oils that are used in aromatherapy. They are extracted or distilled from various parts of plants and trees, where they can be found in special secretory glands or cells. Some plants contain essential oils in their leaves or roots, others in their flowers, fruit, stem, bark, or seeds. Oil of rose, for example, is found in the flower.

EXTRACTING ESSENTIAL OILS

The names of some essential oils give an idea of the diversity of their origins. Some, such as lavender, rosemary, and marjoram, conjure up visions of an English country garden. Others, such as ylang-ylang or sandalwood, evoke images of their more exotic origins.

Essential oils, like wine, have their good years and bad years, and, like any other crop, their quality reflects the quality of the soil. An oil may be therapeutically weaker if it is extracted from a plant grown in poor soil. Some crops, such as lavender, are harvested during the summer, while the flowers used to make essential oil of jasmine are gathered at night when their perfume is more pronounced. It takes many thousands of petals to produce floral oils such as jasmine and rose, because their secretory yield of oil is not high. This is reflected in the price of these oils (they are among the most expensive). Other oils, such as tea tree and eucalyptus, both with a fresh medicinal smell, are more easily produced in larger amounts from a distillation of the leaves or sometimes the stems of their plants. These oils are therefore less expensive.

The most common method of obtaining essential oils from plants is by steam distillation. Plant matter is placed in a still and steam is passed through. Oil particles are carried from the plant matter into another container where the steam is cooled and returned to liquid—now a mixture of water and particles of essential oils from the plant matter. The water separates from the essential oil, which, being lighter, floats on top and is then collected. Steam distillation is the most suitable method of distillation for extracting aromatherapy oils, and, in fact, purists believe that only an oil obtained in this way can be called an essential oil.

But there are other methods of extracting essential oils. With solvent extraction, for example, heated solvents remove oil from the plant material, leaving an odor-laden substance known as a "floral concrete." This method is used for delicate flowers and resins and is more suitable for perfumery than for aromatherapy oils.

Enfleurage, also used for delicate flowers, is a very slow process. Flower petals are placed on glass frames smeared with grease. It takes up to three days for the oil in the petals to be absorbed by the grease. Withered petals are then replaced by fresh ones. The process is repeated many times until the grease is completely saturated with flower oil. The grease is then washed in alcohol to extract the oil.

Expression is a method of extraction used for citrus oils. In the past the oils were squeezed out by hand and collected on sponges. Now this laborious task is performed by machines.

SOME GENERAL PROPERTIES AND USES OF ESSENTIAL OILS

If you imagine that essential oils are rather like vanilla extract that is used in cooking, you will have some idea of their qualities. Obviously, essential oils are much stronger, purer, and more powerful. Although they are called oils, they are not oily like cooking oil and they won't leave a greasy mark on paper or fabric. Their consistency is usually more like that of an alcohol, although some, such as myrrh or benzoin, are thick like runny honey.

Rather in the same way that each of the plants from which they derive has its own flavor and personality, essential oils have their own individual character or "blueprint"—an absolutely unique identity. Essential oils are so potent they need only be used in tiny quantities—usually by the drop—to be beneficial and effective. Each oil has an ingredient list that reads like a laboratory report. Using the sun's energy, plus soil, air, and water, a perfectly balanced cocktail of complex chemicals evolves. It is this combination of elements that gives each oil its individual perfume along with its particular beneficial and healing properties. To date, it is impossible to synthetically produce an essential oil in its exact form.

Essential oils have long been known to contain positive healing, therapeutic, and cosmetic properties. Their use dates back as far as ancient Egypt, and they are widely used today by pharmaceutical and food industries. Peppermint is frequently used in toothpaste, for example, and petitgrain is used in many eaux-de-cologne.

Essential oils are natural antiseptics, some more powerful than others. It has been shown that they can kill airborne viruses, bacteria, and fungi and can neutralize the germs that cause body odor. Unlike some synthetic topical preparations, they help kill germs without harming body tissue when used correctly in dilution.

Some oils, such as chamomile, are analgesic or anti-inflammatory and help reduce aches, pain, and swelling. Others, such as bergamot, have antidepressant qualities and can help alleviate insomnia, anxiety, and mental or physical fatigue. Some oils are very diverse in their properties and uses. Oils such as lavender and tea tree are powerful antiseptics with soothing and healing properties. Tea tree also has excellent antifungal properties and can help conditions such as athlete's foot and yeast infections. Lavender, when diluted in a carrier oil and massaged into the skin, can help relieve labor pains or soothe a headache. It can also help disinfect a bucket of diapers when a few drops are added to a prewash soak. For those new to essential oils, lavender should be their first choice because it has so many different uses.

When using essential oils at home, especially during pregnancy and on the very young, it is important to know the properties of an oil and whether it is sedating, antiseptic, stimulating, or relaxing. All oils have their own properties, but when two or more are mixed together, another unique oil is created and a therapeutic effect or smell can be enhanced. Professional aromatherapists understand the properties of essential oils and can treat individual needs or conditions with their own time-tested recipes. Some of my recipes are found throughout this book.

HOW ESSENTIAL OILS GET INTO THE SKIN

"How can the oil from a fruit or a flower work its way into my body and make me feel good or soothe my pain?" This is one of the questions I am most often asked by my patients. In fact, aromatherapy oils work in two very distinct and different ways: by the sense of smell and by absorption through the skin.

THE SENSE OF SMELL

The sense of smell is often taken for granted, but the human body is capable of registering and recognizing thousands of different smells. Everything has its own smell. Your home, however clean and fresh it may seem to you, will have a recognizable smell to outsiders. How often have you heard people use the phrase, "it doesn't smell like home"?

There are certain smells that we have almost forgotten to recognize. All animals, including humans, produce odoriferous scents called pheromones. Animals have a far more pronounced use of these scents, employing them to warn one another of danger (hence the expression "the smell of fear"), to attract one another sexually, and to mark their territory, as anyone with more than one cat will know. They also use them to identify their own, which is why farmers will skin a dead lamb and use the skin to cover an orphaned one. The mother of the dead lamb will recognize the smell of her offspring and accept this new "baby" as one of her own.

Humans have a smell too and not only what we know as "body odor." Each person has a subtle and individual smell. Your dog will know you by your odor. Likewise, within a few weeks of life, a human baby will learn to recognize the smell of its mother and prefer her company (this includes babies who are bottle-fed). Men and women too are responsive to one another's individual scents. Blonds, brunettes, and redheads apparently have very different smells. The preference some men have for blonds is put down to the fact that blonds apparently exude a smell similar to the smell of babies (small children and babies smell naturally sweet).

Our pheromones change throughout life, and are influenced by factors such as pregnancy, the Pill, hormonal changes, and illness. Diabetics, for example, can exude a smell like acetone, and pneumonia has a dank smell. Babies and children have a different smell than adults. From puberty on, a male could be described as "musky," a scent that women are supposed to find sexually appealing, which is why the musky scent exuded by the male civet cat (now thankfully synthesized) is incorporated into male toiletries.

A woman's pheromones change with her menstrual cycle, becoming sweeter around ovulation. Her own sense of smell is more pronounced then, too, no doubt to seek out a "musky" male. Apparently, men also find women more attractive at this time. It is ironic that we spend a fortune on perfumes and deodorants, applying them liberally before a romantic evening, when the naked, natural smell we possess is more likely to get results. Women who live together have a tendency to menstruate at the same time each month; this is attributed to natural scent regulation, when some subtle glandular odor is picked up. But perhaps the most astonishing example of how overlooked the sense of smell can be is found in recent research into the impressive success of women who fish for trout and salmon (three records established in the 1920s by women anglers have still not been beaten). The theory is that the salmon, which can pick up waterborne chemical messages to a very great degree, are attracted by female pheromones. Apparently, the odors of a man's hand can alarm or repel the salmon, whereas those of a woman's will not.

On a less basic level, smells can trigger both psychological and physiological responses in the body. Aromatic substances, such as essential oils, send out odor molecules. When we breathe these molecules in, receptor cells high in the nose transmit impulses about the odor straight to the olfactory area of the brain, an area closely linked to other systems that control memory, emotions, hormones, sexual feelings, and heart rate. The impulses work quickly, triggering neurochemicals that can stimulate, sedate, relax, or cause euphoria, and bring about changes that can be both psychological and physiological. For example, the Japanese have conducted trials that show that lemon oil vaporized into the air can increase efficiency in the workplace.

These impulses and changes are indications that the sense of smell has powerful and immediate impact on the body; aromatherapy can be effective especially in situations where the heart rate and respiration are affected by fear or anxiety, as in labor. It is hardly surprising that among the essential oils most beneficial for helping stress, anxiety, and depression are the lovely-smelling flower oils such as rose, neroli (from orange blossom), jasmine, and lavender.

In theory, we are subject to a type of aromatherapy every day, anytime a smell triggers a response in the brain. If we unexpectedly catch a hint of a perfume associated with someone we love, for example, it provokes a pleasant, nostalgic feeling. Conversely, a smell we dislike can instantly provoke unpleasant feelings—for example, the smell of carbolic soap or damp paper towels can transport us back to our school days. In *Remembrance of Things Past,* it is the aroma of a madeleine cake that takes Proust back to his childhood. Smells can alert us to danger (such as the smell of smoke or something burning), warn us to avoid certain actions (such as eating food or milk that has gone sour), stimulate digestion, and even make us more alert.

THE SKIN

The skin is the body's largest organ. It could be described as the packaging that keeps us warm, stops rain from getting in, and stops our insides from falling out. But it is a lot more than simple "wrapping paper." It acts as an outer warning system, relaying messages to the brain about our environment by means of temperature, pain, touch, and so forth, and reflects the inner body by showing age and state of health.

Some people find it hard to believe that our skin is anything other than a thick waterproof covering. To a certain extent this is true. We don't absorb bathwater, for example; neither do we absorb heavy, thick mineral oils, such as petroleum jelly, which leave a greasy layer on the skin. But it is possible for the skin to allow certain substances to filter through if their molecular structure is small enough.

The skin is one of the body's organs of elimination. We lose sweat and other soluble wastes through the skin. In the same way we can let things out, we can also let things in. Doctors are increasingly administering medications, such as antiangina drugs and hormone replacement therapy (HRT), by applying them to the skin, which means they bypass the digestive system and, in turn, are kinder to the body's internal organs.

Whether applied to the skin in a carrier oil or used in the bath, the tiny molecular structure of an essential oil enables it to pass through the skin. It travels via the hair follicles, diffusing into the bloodstream, or is taken into the lymphatic and extracellular fluids, at which point the organic, therapeutic ingredients of the essential oil are broken down and used by the body for the intended purpose, such as, for example, when you have massaged on chamomile oil for its pain-relieving properties.

It can take anywhere from twenty minutes to seven hours for oils applied to the skin to be fully absorbed into the body. The amount of time varies according to the amount of body fat (the more there is, the longer it takes), which is why aromatherapists request that clients not shower or bathe for at least seven hours after a treatment to ensure that none of the oil is washed off.

After performing their healing functions on the body, essential oils are eliminated along with all the body's other wastes, such as sweat and urine. The body is left in a healthier state, without any of the side effects modern drugs can cause.

3

A History of
Essential Oils

The way to health is to have an aromatic bath
and a scented massage every day.

Hippocrates

"A woman lies relaxing while skilled hands rub warm, scented oils
rhythmically over her body. . . ." This description of a woman of the
twenty-first century enjoying a massage could apply equally well to an
Egyptian woman of around 3000 years B.C.E. Although aromatherapy
may seem like a relatively new branch of complementary medicine, the
practice of using oils for perfuming, healing, and religious ceremonies
can be traced back thousands of years.

In the 1920s, when archaeologists uncovered the tombs of the
pharaohs, they discovered jars of fragrant oils, still with a faint aroma
even after thousands of years. Egyptian mummies were so well preserved
because the resins and essential oils used for embalmment contained
antibacterial and antiseptic properties that prevented putrification and
decay. Essential oils of cedarwood, myrrh, galbanum clove, and nutmeg
were impregnated in bandages wrapped around the mummies.

In ancient Egypt it was the priests who prescribed medicines and
who knew the power of oils, which they also used to alter moods in

religious ceremonies. The oils used were most likely not distilled (see chapter 2) but rather were produced either by dropping aromatic plants or resin gums into animal fat, which was then left in the sun until impregnated by the scent, or by steeping the plant material in olive or sesame oil. The method of distilling oils from plants, in basically the manner that we use today with essential oils, was reputed to have been discovered by an Arab physician, Avicenna, in the tenth century.

There are frequent references to essential oils in the Bible. In Exodus 20:26, for example, Moses was instructed by God to take fine spices of liquid myrrh, fragrant cinnamon, cane, cassia, and olive oil and blend them into a sacred anointing oil. In the Book of Esther, virgins chosen for the harem had to complete twelve months of beauty treatments specially prescribed for the women—six months with oil of myrrh and six with perfumes and cosmetics—before being taken to the king.

The infamous Cleopatra apparently knew of the aphrodisiacal charms of oils and seduced Antony after bathing in jasmine with her room scattered with rose petals. Along with so much else of their culture, the Egyptians passed their knowledge and love of aromatic perfumes to the Greeks, who in turn advanced this knowledge by looking at the medicinal value of plants and perfecting the art of steeping flower petals in carrier oils, such as olive oil, for medicinal and cosmetic use.

During this period of history, Greek physicians, such as Hippocrates, Galen, and Dioscorides, left their mark on the world through their writing and research into plants. Many of their findings have been confirmed by twentieth-century research. Hippocrates, now known as the father of medicine and whose name is given to the oath doctors take today, was the first physician to observe the progression of an illness and to use that knowledge when treating the next case he encountered. He was aware of the antibacterial properties of certain plants and once, during a plague in Athens, implored the populace to burn these plants in the streets so that the aromatic fumes could protect them.

Galen, physician to the gladiators, discovered that he could mix vegetable oil with beeswax and water to produce a cream that was soothing and that kept the skin soft. He had, in fact, made the first "cold cream." Greek soldiers, when going into battle, probably carried the first first-aid kit—a small bag containing myrrh, which helped heal their wounds. Myrrh is still used for healing purposes today. I find it excellent for treating stubborn leg ulcers.

At the height of the Roman empire great emphasis was placed on the benefits of bathing. The rich and fashionable had magnificent bathing areas built into their homes, areas large enough to hold parties, and indulged in long rituals of soaking in warm water. They used oils such as lavender (its botanical name, *Lavandula officinalis,* comes from the Latin verb *lavare,* meaning "to wash") to perfume the water and followed these luxurious baths with massages, again using scented oils. They also carried out what we know today as a very efficient way of removing dirt and dead skin cells. A mixture of pumice and olive oil was rubbed over the body, then scraped off with a narrow scraper called a strigil, leaving the skin soft and clean. Lesser mortals would, of course, attend the public baths.

While Rome bathed, its armies marched; with them they carried herbs and oils for medicinal and culinary needs. Where they invaded they planted seeds. Many of what we regard today as typical English garden herbs, such as lavender, lovage, parsley, and fennel, are legacies from the Romans.

After the fall of the Roman Empire, teachings and books written about aromatics reached the Arab world. It was there that essential oil of rose was first distilled, and with it came rose water, which is widely used even now in Middle Eastern countries, especially in cooking. Trade routes flourished between East and West, bringing to Europe spices and aromatics from the East, including sandalwood from India. The perfumes of Arabia became much-sought-after substances. While the Romans had taken many herb seeds to foreign countries, the Crusaders took exotic perfumes and essential oils back to their own lands along with the knowledge of how to distill them. The essential oil trade had truly begun.

During the Middle Ages the use of herbs and aromatic oils was commonplace. Cooking was performed with liberal amounts of herbs and spices, not only to enhance flavor but to mask the taste of putrid meat. There was also widespread knowledge of the medicinal and antiseptic properties of plants.

In the larger, wealthier homes there would have been a still room—a place especially set aside for working with herbs and plants. It was there that all kinds of aromatic recipes were made, including ointments, strong herbal waters, and basic medicinal potions. Cloth sachets filled with dry herbs were made to lay among clothes (as protection against moths) and linens. Mattresses and pillows, too, were stuffed with sweet-smelling herbs and flowers.

The Middle Ages were notorious for the unsanitary conditions in which the average person lived. Aromatic oils were used not just for pleasure and cleanliness—often they were the only means available to wage war on disease and pain. Plants such as lavender, hyssop, thyme, and mint were strewn on floors to help disguise the strong smells that resulted from the lack of sanitation facilities and the lack of personal hygiene. Powerful herbs such as thyme and rosemary were hung in bunches around the house or burned on the fire when illness threatened—the inhabitants quickly learned that wherever strong scents lingered, illness was less likely to rear its head.

During the late sixteenth and early seventeenth centuries, many herbal texts were written by physicians and apothecaries such as Nicholas Culpeper, John Gerard, and John Parkinson. These texts praised and detailed herbal remedies and cataloged strange new plants that were beginning to arrive from the New World. The trades of apothecary and perfumer flourished, and in times of epidemics and plagues, it was the people from these professions who, working on a daily basis with essential oils, frequently escaped illness.

By the 1880s chemists were discovering how to quickly and cheaply synthesize equivalents to many healing herbs and other plants. Thus the modern pharmaceutical industry was born. As medical science advanced, herbal medicine was viewed with an increasingly suspicious eye. Although doctors used essential oils until the latter part of the nineteenth century as a routine part of their medicine kits, interest in using these oils for general medical purposes faded and they began to be used for lesser purposes—as flavorings and in the perfume industry.

Research into the properties of essential oils continued, however. The first documented laboratory research into their antiseptic properties was carried out in Paris in 1887 by Dr. Chamberland. He confirmed, as did others after him, that essential oils could kill airborne viruses, bacteria, and fungi when sprayed into the air. Despite this important information, however, the doctors and chemists of the day preferred the new synthetic types of medication.

By the beginning of the twentieth century, essential oils were pushed back onto laboratory shelves, even though they had proved their practical worth countless times over the centuries. Interest in essential oils was reawakened by the French chemist Rene Gattefosse. His original interest in essential oils began purely by chance. During an experiment in his laboratory, Gattefosse burned his hand and plunged it into the nearest liquid, which happened to be lavender oil. His burned hand rapidly became less inflamed and painless, and the subsequent rate of healing was extraordinarily fast. This prompted Gattefosse to research essential oils and their medical application, particularly in dermatology. In 1937 he published a book that he called *Aromatherapy*—a name that would open up a whole new era for essential oils.

Inspired by Gattefosse's research papers, a French army doctor, John Valnet, began his own clinical research using essential oils as antiseptics on soldiers he treated in the Indo-China war. He was so impressed by the results of his research that he used essential oils to treat war veterans with psychological problems. He has since written many books and articles on aromatherapy, including *The Practice of Aromatherapy,* which is now a standard text for every professional aromatherapist.

The practice of aromatherapy as we know it today—combining essential oils with massage for health, beauty, and well-being—was started by the Austrian biochemist Marguerite Maury. Her husband was a homeopathic doctor, and both of them took a great interest in all forms of alternative medicine. Based on her knowledge of essential oils, Maury undertook a program of research, demonstrating the effectiveness of the oils when they are absorbed through the skin. She was particularly interested in their healing and rejuvenating properties. In 1962, and again in 1967, Maury received major awards for her work. As well as lecturing about and sharing her knowledge of essential oils, she opened several clinics in Europe, including one in London. In 1961 Maury published the book *Le Capital "Jeunesse,"* which has now been reprinted and is currently available in English as *The Secret of Life and Youth* (C.W. Daniel Company Ltd., 1989).

THE HISTORY OF ESSENTIAL OILS IN CHILDBIRTH

In the Western world the use of plant oils in childbirth, just as in general medicine, has come full circle. Until the middle of the nineteenth century, women usually gave birth with other women helping them, most likely women from their own families, who had had children themselves or local women who were experienced in labor or who had witnessed many deliveries. Normally, men were only called upon for their strength, to physically assist a mother who was weak after a long labor. This was often at the expense of both mother and baby, unless it was a shepherd who was used to birthing difficult lambs, in which case the mother's chances of survival were higher.

There were no drugs to ease labor pains, so these early midwives used the only things they knew could help: aromatic plants and other substances. Recipes and knowledge used to heal and deaden pain were handed down from mother to daughter, along with panaceas for many other ailments. One of the substances used in childbirth was ergot, a cereal fungus that helps the uterus contract. A derivative, ergometrine, is still used today in the injection given immediately after birth to help the uterus contract and expel the placenta.

The Church disagreed that women should be relieved of pain during childbirth. According to the Bible, women were supposed to "bring forth children in sorrow." During the Middle Ages these views, along with the politics of the day, often encouraged women to obtain valuable knowledge of the pain-relieving power of aromatics and herbal remedies that the Church associated with witchcraft.

Medicine advanced with the discovery of "laughing gas" in 1772. The practice of using remedies administered by women gradually faded as the use of drugs increased. Substances such as chloroform and morphine were used along with scopolamine (known as "twilight sleep" because the mother became nearly unconscious). Men became the authorities on drugs—and thus childbirth—while midwives were considered second-class care providers. Women became conditioned to believe that birth meant pain and fear and that labor and delivery meant giving birth flat on their backs while they were most likely heavily sedated (all, of course, purely for the convenience of the male doctor).

During the 1930s Dr. Grantly Dick-Read observed this fear of childbirth in his patients and he and others, such as Fernand Lamaze, recognized that childbirth without conditioned fear was possible and that mothers could participate in and enjoy birth without interference from drugs. By the late 1940s a new era had opened up for women, an era that encouraged the use of breathing methods, relaxation, and massage as aids to a pain-controlled labor. Aromatherapy has also become a highly acceptable form of treatment over the last decade. Women can be in control of their pain and emotions using the time-tested healing powers of aromatics. They also now have a choice about how they give birth; even for those in favor of modern methods of pain relief, aromatherapy and massage can still play an important part in their labor, as backup to conventional treatment.

In many hospitals nurses who have taken aromatherapy courses are now using essential oils, sometimes in labor wards. At the birth unit at St. John's and St. Elizabeth's Hospital in London, one midwife told me that "aromatherapy is a way of life here." It is one of their patients' first choices for pain relief in labor and is used postpartum and for baby care. Essential oils are also used at the delivery suite and postpartum wards of Hinchingbrooke Hospital in Huntingdon, England, where mid-wives are happy for mothers-to-be to bring their own essential oils for labor or to use those supplied by the midwives. There has recently been a trial study at this hospital testing lavender oil versus conventional treatment for the relief of postpartum perineal pain; the results have yet to be published. At last, aromatherapy seems to be gaining the status it deserves for labor and childbirth.

4

How to Use Essential Oils

Essential oils can be worked into the body in several different ways. The most common and safe ways of using them are listed below. Recommended oils and recipes for the various methods are included in the relevant chapters.

MASSAGE

Massage is helpful for relieving stress and tension, for aiding relaxation, for easing aching muscles, and for general pain relief as well as for improving skin tone and general well-being. In aromatherapy massage, the essential oils are added to a carrier oil, such as almond or jojoba, before being applied to the skin.

BODY MASSAGE

Pour a small amount of preprepared massage oil in the palms of the hands (½–1 teaspoonful will do a back or leg adequately, unless the person receiving the massage has very hairy or dry skin). Massage gently into the body. Always massage toward the heart. Don't massage near varicose veins (glide around them), on hot, swollen joints, or when a fever is present. See chapter 7 for full instructions on body massage.

FOOT MASSAGE

A foot massage is wonderful for relieving tension and to revive and re-energize a tired body. It's also bliss for swollen or aching feet. I guarantee that once you get the hang of it, the person receiving the foot rub will beg for more. Spread the preprepared oil all over one foot and around the ankle. With hands cupped around the foot and fingers steadying the front of the foot, use the thumbs to make circular pressures on the sole. Gently squeeze and press the foot as though you were trying to make it into a pliable piece of dough. Repeat with the other foot.

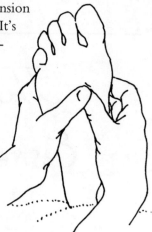

FACIAL MASSAGE

A facial massage will help care for any type of skin in every condition, both during and after pregnancy.

Apply the preprepared oil very sparingly to the face and neck at night after cleansing. Always use gentle upward movements to apply the oil (to reverse the effects of gravity). Try not to drag the skin. If you are massaging someone's face, ask them to remove their contact lenses. See chapter 13 for full instructions and recipes for facial massage oils.

AROMATIC BATHS

Aromatic baths are an important part of aromatherapy. Depending upon the oils used, they can be detoxifying, refreshing, and reviving when taken in the morning, or sedating, calming, and soothing when taken in the evening. They help promote a restful night's sleep if taken just before bed and are helpful for reducing aches and pains.

For an aromatic bath during pregnancy, add 2–4 drops of the chosen essential oil to a warm bath (never too hot). Swish the water around to disperse the oil. Relax and soak in the bath for ten to fifteen minutes to enjoy the aroma and let the oils do their work.

SITZ BATH OR BIDET

Both a sitz bath and a bidet are used for washing and soothing the hips and genital area (particularly useful for just after childbirth). A sitz bath can be improvised by filling an ordinary bath with enough warm water to just cover the lower abdomen.

Add 2 drops of the chosen essential oil to a sitz bath or bidet. Mix the water well before stepping in. Soak for five to ten minutes.

CHILDREN'S BATHS

Children can benefit from aromatic baths as much as adults, but smaller quantities of oil should be used. Even the mildest of essential oils must always be very well diluted to avoid getting any drops of undiluted oil on the child's hands, which could then be rubbed into the eyes or mouth. Children also have very delicate skin that can be easily irritated.

The essential oils should be diluted in ½–1 tablespoon (10–20 milliliters) of whole milk. Goat's milk can be used if the child is allergic to cow's milk. Count out the drops (see below for quantities) into a small bowl, add the milk, stir well, and add to the bathwater.

I recommend using no more than the following amounts of essential oil:

- For children five to twelve years of age, add 2–4 drops of essential oil to the milk.

- For children two to five years of age, add 1–2 drops of essential oil to the milk.

- For babies over three months and very young children, add just 1 drop.

I don't recommend essential oils in the bath for babies under three months, and even older children should not have them as a matter of course.

FOOTBATHS

Add 2–3 drops of the chosen essential oil to a bowl of hot water. Soak the feet for ten to twenty minutes.

SHOWERS

Essential oils can be used in the shower. The best way to use them is to wash as normal, then add 2–3 drops of your chosen essential oil to a sponge or washcloth and rub it over the body while standing under the water and breathing the vapors.

COMPRESSES

Compresses are wonderful for treating labor pain. They are also useful for muscular aches and pains, sprains, or bruises and to help reduce pain in general.

For acute inflammation, such as headaches, swellings, sprains, wounds, and so forth, use a cold compress. For chronic pain, such as backache, muscular pain, labor pain, earache, and so forth, use a hot compress. For wounds or infected boils, the water should be previously boiled and cotton wool or sterile gauze should be used as a compress.

Add 2–4 drops of essential oil to 8 ounces (240 milliliters) of water (either hot or cold according to which compress is needed). Agitate to mix the oils. Take a small cloth, washcloth, or towel and lay it on top of the water so that the oils are picked up on the underside. Lay the cloth on the affected part. Cover with a small, dry towel and leave in place until the cold compress has warmed to body temperature or the hot compress has lost heat. Renew as required.

INHALATIONS

Inhalations are used to clear congestion that comes with colds and sinusitis. They can be extremely effective in unblocking the nose and helping relieve the nasal passages.

STEAM INHALATIONS

Steam inhalations are not suitable for asthmatics (they may, of course, use essential oils in the bath) or for children under ten years of age, as they can be quite dangerous. It is also not safe for a small child to sit over a bowl of hot water. Children over ten years old should be attended at all times if they have an inhalation, and they should only inhale the steam for a few minutes. In fact, if they have a cold, it is better to sniff the oils on a tissue or have the oil vaporized in a room near them. Smaller children can have the same oils in the bath in a low dilution (1–2 drops only). Or, for sniffly babies, the oils can be used in a special room vaporizer.

To a bowl of very hot (but not boiling) water, add 2–4 drops of the essential oil. Cover your head with a small dry towel (if you choose to), lean over the bowl, and breathe in the vapor for one to five minutes.

USING A TISSUE OR HANDKERCHIEF

Add 1 drop of essential oil to a tissue or clean handkerchief, and sniff when needed. This is a very handy method of using essential oils if you have a cold, but it is also quite comforting postpartum if you can't have essential oils beside the bed in the hospital. It's also very useful during labor.

TO PERFUME ROOMS AND PURIFY THE AIR

Essential oils can be used not only to add a delicious and relaxing aroma to a room but also—depending upon the oil used, of course—to dispel bacteria and remove unwanted smells. There are many different ways of using essential oils to scent rooms.

WITH HOT WATER

Add 2–6 drops of essential oil to a bowl of hot water. Let this stand in the room.

WITH A PLANT ATOMIZER

With an appropriate essential oil, using an atomizer is an ideal way to dispel bacteria when there is illness in the house. Fill a plant atomizer with 8 ounces (240 milliliters) of water. Add 6 drops of essential oil. Spray this mixture around the room.

IN A BURNER

A burner can be bought at most health food stores. Always make sure that the bowl of the burner is washed regularly to avoid the buildup of sticky, caramelized oils on the base.

Fill the top bowl of the burner with water. Add 2–3 drops of essential oil. Burn for as long as you choose—perhaps an hour—then extinguish the candle and allow the aroma to waft around the room.

ON A LIGHTBULB RING

Lightbulb rings are available at most health food stores. Follow the maker's instructions for using lightbulb rings. Some are solid round rings and the oil can be dropped straight onto them; others have a reservoir inside into which the oil can be dropped straight or diluted with water.

Use 2–3 drops of essential oil and place the ring onto a lightbulb (in a table lamp is best). The heat from the bulb will warm the oil and disperse the aroma throughout the room.

IN A DIFFUSER

Diffusers are available at major department stores and pharmacies. Follow the maker's instructions for using diffusers (they vary). Make sure you purchase one with a bowl that is easily wiped clean; otherwise the diffuser will have a buildup of different essential oils on the base of the bowl.

ON COTTON BALLS

Cotton balls can be used in the rooms of babies or small children, but take great care and make sure the cotton ball is placed where it cannot possibly be reached. If in doubt, don't use this method.

Add 2–6 drops of the chosen essential oil to a cotton ball. Lodge behind the warm part of a radiator.

BY SCENTING A FIRE

In wintertime it is wonderful to place just 1 drop of essential oil onto each log just *before* placing it on the fire. Remember, though, that essential oils are quite volatile and inflammable, so don't drop the oils straight into the fire.

IN A VACUUM CLEANER

A vacuum cleaner can be used to freshen the entire house or to remove unpleasant smells. Add 3–4 drops of essential oil to a couple of cotton balls. Pop them into the vacuum cleaner bag and they will freshen each room you vacuum. The aroma can linger for quite some time.

A WORD OF CAUTION

Essential oils are powerful and need to be diluted before applying directly to the skin. They should always be used either in a carrier oil, or mixed with water, or added by the drop to creams and lotions. If they are not diluted, some oils, such as the citrus oils, could cause soreness and irritation.

However, as in all things in life, there are exceptions to this rule. Two oils—lavender and tea tree—can be used directly on the skin but only in very small quantities, literally by the drop. Always follow recipe directions or use them as directed by a qualified aromatherapist. Even so, some people with very sensitive skin may be unable to tolerate undiluted forms of these two mild oils.

Essential oils should never be taken by mouth—they are far too strong for the delicate lining of the alimentary tract.

PATCH TESTING

If you have sensitive skin or suffer from eczema, dermatitis, or allergies, such as hayfever, you may wish to consult an aromatherapist before using any essential oils (see Appendix 1 to find one in your area). She or he may recommend doing a patch test.

❧ Add 2 drops of the essential oil you want to test to ½ tablespoon (10 milliliters) of a carrier oil.

❧ Smear a little on the inside of the elbow. There is no need to cover it. Leave the area unwashed for twenty-four hours.

❧ If any redness or itching occurs, do not use that oil—you may have an allergy to it.

If you are prone to allergic reactions from nut or vegetable oils, you may also have to test the carrier oil. It is obviously better to test the carrier oil before you test the essential oil. Follow the above procedure by rubbing a smear of the carrier oil you wish to test on the inside of your elbow. Leave for twenty-four hours. If there is no reaction (such as redness or irritation), proceed to test the essential oil. If there is an adverse reaction, try the procedure again with another carrier oil.

5

A Guide to Essential Oils

There is currently a vast range of essential oils available in stores but only certain ones should be used during pregnancy: those that are gentle and soothing. Stimulating oils should never be used because their effects are not particularly desirable during pregnancy, (for a full list of oils to be avoided during pregnancy see pages 40–41).

ESSENTIAL OILS OF GREATEST USE DURING PREGNANCY

LAVENDER
Lavandula officinalis: **from the lavender flower**

Lavender oil is known as the "great all-arounder" because it has so many uses. Anyone new to aromatherapy would do well to invest in some lavender oil. It is antibiotic and antiseptic and good for pimples, scrapes, and minor burns. Used in skin creams, it can help cell renewal and minimize scarring. It soothes insect bites, fights off infections, relieves headaches, and eases muscular aches and pains. In pregnancy lavender oil is particularly useful for soothing aching backs, legs, and ligaments.

Among the many qualities of lavender oil are its relaxing and antidepressant properties. It has a mild sedative action so it helps insomnia, and it is a wonderful oil to use in the bath at the end of the day or to scent the room before sleep. It is, in fact, less an oil than a medicine chest in a bottle. It is one of two oils (the other being tea tree) that is gentle enough to be used in small quantities directly on the skin.

A smear of lavender oil applied to a minor burn is the perfect first-aid treatment (after plunging the burn into cold running water if possible). If this oil is used at intervals during the day, it will help remove the sting, stop infection, and minimize scarring.

Use for baths, massages, room fresheners, and facial oils. (See the note on lavender oil under "Essential Oil Safety" on page 39.)

MANDARIN
Citrus nobilis: from the rind of the mandarin

Mandarin has very similar properties to tangerine—calming, gentle, and cheery—but it has a slightly fresher smell. It is used in baths because its gentle tonic effects help relieve fatigue. In leg and ankle massages, mandarin can ease fluid retention.

Use for baths, massages, and room fresheners.

NEROLI
Citrus aurantium: from the flowers of the bitter orange tree

An absolutely heavenly oil, neroli is also diabolically expensive but worth every penny because the aroma is so exquisite. It makes a wonderful facial oil, good for dry or sensitive skin, and will help regenerate skin cells. It is one of the very best oils to use for nervous tension (I call it the "antipanic oil") because it is so calming and relaxing. It is rumored to have aphrodisiac qualities and is also a deeply peaceful oil. Neroli is excellent to use during pregnancy for its ability to promote healthy skin cells.

Use for baths, massages, room fresheners, and facial oils.

PETITGRAIN
Citrus aurantium: from the leaves and twigs
of the bitter orange tree

Petitgrain has similar properties to neroli—calming and soothing—but it is slightly less sedating with a fresher perfume, so it can be used as a cheaper alternative to neroli. It makes a lovely room scenter. It is particularly helpful for dealing with depression, either during the pregnancy or postpartum. A very special massage mix can be made using all three oils from the orange tree: petitgrain from the leaves and twigs, neroli from the flowers, and orange from the fruit. Blended together they make what I call a "total balance" oil, a very whole treatment that I use for those who are depressed (see page 88 for the recipe).

Use for baths, massages, and room fresheners.

TANGERINE
Citrus reticulata: **from the rind of the tangerine**

A nice, happy oil and my favorite pregnancy oil, tangerine has a wonderfully uplifting smell. It helps prevent stretch marks, which makes it excellent to use in massage during pregnancy. Tangerine is a beneficial oil to use when a tonic is needed—it is calming, gentle, and good for the nerves and skin. Because it is so mild, it is also a good oil to use for children and the elderly. Supposedly rich in vitamin C, tangerine is well known as a tonic for upset stomachs.

Use in baths, massages, and room fresheners.

YLANG-YLANG
Canaga odorata: **from the flowers**
of the tropical ylang-ylang tree

Ylang-ylang oil is very exotic and famed for its perfume. It has relaxing, restoring, and aphrodisiac properties and can even help lower high blood pressure. It can also be used to help those who are tense and worried and is good used in a bath blend.

Use in baths, massages, and room fresheners.

ESSENTIAL OILS FOR LIMITED USE DURING PREGNANCY

The following oils can be used as all-over massage oils but are not recommended during pregnancy. They are better added to gels and massage oils to be used on specific areas, such as aching legs.

CYPRESS

Cupressus sempervirens: from the evergreen tree

Cypress oil has astringent qualities and is a gentle diuretic. I use it after the fifth month of pregnancy because it is particularly helpful, in a cooling lotion or gel, for varicose veins. Added to a bath, lotion, or wash, it can help hemorrhoids. Its gentle diuretic action can assist in decongesting fluid retention in heavy, aching legs and swollen ankles.

Use after the fifth month of pregnancy, in local application gels, oils, and washes.

GERANIUM

Pelargonium graveolens: from the geranium plant

Geranium oil is known as an all-around balancer because it re-establishes equilibrium. It is a very strong oil and is best avoided as a body massage in pregnancy. Geranium is astringent, refreshing, and relaxing and has a lovely aroma. I use it after the fifth month of pregnancy for the wonderful relief it gives to tired and aching legs—it is good for poor circulation.

Use in room fresheners and after the fifth month of pregnancy in local massage gels, footbaths, and oils.

LEMON

Citrus limonum: from the rind of the lemon

Lemon has a fresh, sharp citrus smell. It is refreshing, cooling, and antiseptic, and it aids the circulation. During pregnancy it can be used in a burner for morning sickness and in a local massage oil or gel for varicose veins.

Use in local massage gels or oils or as a room freshener.

SANDALWOOD

Santalum album: from the sandalwood tree

Sandalwood is an exotic and relaxing oil and an excellent facial oil for dry or sensitive skin. It can be particularly helpful for urinary infections during pregnancy.

Use in baths and for skin care.

TEA TREE
Melaleuca alternifolia: from the tropical tea tree

An incredibly useful essential oil, tea tree (along with lavender) is one of the essential oils mild enough to be used in small quantities directly on the skin. It is usually used to treat cuts and wounds and is an excellent antifungal oil, useful for cuts, pimples, and wounds and as an inhalation for colds. It can be used to deal with yeast infections during pregnancy.

Use in local-application washes and creams.

CARRIER OILS

All essential oils are blended and diluted into a carrier oil before using for massage. Only a very few drops of essential oil are needed in proportion to the carrier oil, rather in the same way that only a pinch of herbs or spices is needed in cooking. Carrier oils in aromatherapy are usually cold-pressed vegetable oils, rich in vitamins, proteins, and minerals. They literally "carry" the essential oil into the body and help lubricate the skin so the aromatherapist's hands can massage without dragging.

If you have very sensitive skin, you may be allergic to certain carrier oils. Try a patch test first (see page 31).

The following carrier oils are ones I have found most suitable for use during pregnancy, postpartum, and for babies.

SWEET ALMOND OIL
from almond nut kernels

Rich in vitamins, sweet almond oil is particularly good for dry skin. It is light and easy to absorb and blends well with other oils. It can be used for face or body massage and is the most suitable oil to use for baby massage.

Use for face, body, and babies.

AVOCADO OIL
from the avocado flesh

Avocado is a very nourishing oil. It is usually mixed with other carrier oils because it tends to be a little too heavy to use alone, but it penetrates easily and deeply and is therefore excellent for keeping skin supple and helping prevent stretch marks. Avocado oil is rich in protein and in vitamins A, D, and E.

Use for face and body.

GRAPESEED OIL
from the grape seed

Grapeseed oil is popular for massage because it is light and nonsticky, and it usually doesn't provoke allergies. It is widely available, even in supermarkets, but it is best to buy a high-quality grapeseed oil, preferably in a glass bottle.

Use for face and body.

JOJOBA
pronounced ho-ho-ba: from the beans of the shrub

Jojoba, more a wax than an oil, has healing and deep moisturizing properties. It penetrates the skin easily and, when used as a facial oil, mixes with and dissolves sebum and unclogs pores, which makes it an excellent oil to use on skin that is prone to acne.

Jojoba is good for all skin types. It can be used by those with sensitive skin (particularly if the skin is also dry and wrinkly) and sparingly by those with eczema. It makes a good facial moisturizer— I use it as a base in all my facial massage oils—but is also excellent to use as a baby oil, especially where there is chapped skin.

Use for face, body, and baby.

WHEATGERM OIL
from the wheat "germ" or grain

Wheatgerm is a very heavy, strong-smelling oil rich in vitamin E, which is good for people with dry or lined skin. It is very helpful in preventing stretch marks and for healing scars left by pimples, wounds, or burns. One of nature's natural antioxidants, wheatgerm will help preserve and prolong the life of any blended mix of essential oils and carrier oils, such as a massage oil mix, if it makes up 10 percent of the mix—that is, in a 1½-ounce (50-milliliter) bottle, add 1 teaspoon (5 milliliters) of wheatgerm to 10 teaspoons (45 milliliters) of sweet almond oil. Wheatgerm is not an oil I use, however, because it tends to have a fishy smell and must not be used by those who have an allergy to wheat.

Use for face and body.

CALENDULA
Calendula officinalis: from macerated marigold flowers

Calendula oil is very healing, has antiseptic properties, and is good for inflamed or delicate skin. I recommend using it in a cream for sore or cracked nipples and for babies, when it comprises 10 percent of a mixture with sweet almond oil, to clean around sore areas caused by diaper rash.

ALOE VERA
from the leaves of the plant

Aloe vera is a gelatinous substance that is frequently used in creams and hair conditioners. It has moisturizing properties and can help soothe burned or irritated skin. When incorporated into a gel, aloe makes a good medium to which essential oils may be added. The oils can be blended with aloe vera either on their own or with other carrier oils. When buying aloe gel, make sure it contains a high percentage of aloe vera.

Use for face, body, and baby.

APRICOT KERNEL
Prunus armeniaca

A light-textured and nourishing oil with virtually no odor, apricot is an ideal carrier medium for baby massage and for anyone who has, or is concerned about, nut allergies. It is suitable for delicate, sensitive, and prematurely aged skins.

Use for face, body, and baby.

OLIVE OIL
Olea europa

Olive oil is heavy with a strong odor and a sticky feeling. Although it is not recommended for an all-over body massage, its soothing properties do have a beneficial action on dry, dehydrated, or inflamed skin. Use it to nourish dry elbows, hands, and heels.

Newborns frequently have dry peeling skin on their legs and feet. A little olive oil massaged gently into the skin can help smooth any dry areas.

Use for face, body, and baby.

MIXING THE OILS

Because most essential oils are far too strong to use directly on the skin, they are diluted with carrier oils for massage. Several different carrier oils are often mixed together to form the base for a massage oil.

MIXING THE BASE OIL

The best base oil for a pregnancy massage is a blend of 80 percent sweet almond oil and 20 percent avocado oil. This base oil can be kept ready for use. Whenever you wish to mix an oil for massage, add the desired essential oil.

Pour 2 tablespoons (40 milliliters) of sweet almond oil and ½ tablespoon (10 milliliters) of avocado oil into a clean, dry bottle. Mix well.

ADDING ESSENTIAL OILS

As a general guide use only 1 drop of essential oil to every ¼ tablespoon (approximately 4–5 milliliters) of base oil. The quantities given below are ideal to use for pregnancy massage oils. Don't be tempted to exceed the stated amount of essential oil, especially for oils to be used during pregnancy or for babies. Some essential oils come out of the dropper very, very fast, so, before making up your blend, practice with the dropper. This way the blend won't be spoiled.

- To 2½ tablespoons (50 milliliters) of base oil, add 10–12 drops of essential oil.

- To 5 tablespoons (100 milliliters) of base oil, add 20–25 drops of essential oil.

ESSENTIAL OIL SAFETY

OILS TO AVOID WHEN PREGNANT

I always use, and advise my clients to use, very limited amounts of essential oils during pregnancy. I have treated many pregnant women and all of them have sailed happily and aromatically through their pregnancies. Nevertheless, as with all things taken in by or applied to the body during this time, you should be extra cautious, even to the point of being overcautious.

Aromatherapists advise that certain essential oils not be used during pregnancy. Some are considered too stimulating or too strong for a pregnant woman's vulnerable system and may cross the placental barrier. Others, known as emmenagogic oils, can stimulate menstruation and should be avoided, particularly in early pregnancy. You may find that some aromatherapists recommend avoiding these oils only during the first three to five months of pregnancy. I feel it is safer if they are avoided altogether. Enjoy the ones that you can safely use.

The only exceptions I make to this rule are lavender, chamomile, and cypress. Although it has diuretic and emmenagogic properties, lavender is so very mild that it can be used in early pregnancy. However, both lavender and chamomile should be avoided if there has been any abnormal bleeding. I use cypress in later pregnancy for local application to treat hemorrhoids.

I am often asked about the effects of using one of the oils that is not recommended, say before a woman knew she was pregnant. Don't panic if this has happened to you. The amount of oil used during a massage, for example, is quite low. It is the continuous and indiscriminate use of these oils that causes concern. Discontinue using any oils that are not recommended, and inform your aromatherapist as soon as you even suspect you may be pregnant.

Before you buy any essential oils for pregnancy, familiarize yourself with the gentle ones suitable for pregnant women and carefully follow the recipes given in this book. Remember, the quantities have been very thoroughly worked out and when used in the proper way, they are highly beneficial.

One last thing: I am frequently asked by patients if they can continue to use the herb form of essential oils that are not recommended. Essential oils are much stronger and more concentrated than the herb or plant from which they are derived, so even if you are advised not to use certain essential oils, you can still use the herb. Oils such as basil, rosemary, or mint should be avoided while pregnant, but there is no harm whatsoever in using these herbs when cooking.

Oils to avoid when pregnant

Angelica	Hyssop	Peppermint
Aniseed	Jasmine	Rosemary
Basil	Juniper	Savory
Camphor	Lovage	Sage

Cedarwood	Melissa	Spanish Marjoram
Clary Sage	Myrrh	Sweet Marjoram
Clove	Marjoram	Tarragon
Cinnamon	Origanum	Thyme
Fennel	Parsley	

There are so many oils available these days that there are bound to be some I have not mentioned in this book. Don't buy an oil you have never heard of or read about, and if you have any doubts about an oil, leave it well alone until you can find out full and reliable information about it.

Oils That Should Never be Used in Aromatherapy

Arnica	Jaborandi Leaf	Southernwood
Armoise	Mustard	Tansy
Baldo Leaf	Pennyroyal	Thuga
Bitter Almond	Rue	Wormwood
Calamus	Sassafras	Wintergreen
Horseradish	Savin	

A SPECIAL WORD OF CAUTION

If you suffer from epilepsy or any sensitivity of the central nervous system, always consult an aromatherapist and let her or him advise you about your choice of essential oils. Some oils, if used indiscriminately or without care, could aggravate your condition or even trigger an attack. Do not use fennel, hyssop, sage, wormwood, or rosemary.

If you suffer from asthma, eczema, dermatitis, or any other allergies, aromatherapy can certainly be of help, but ask the advice of an aromatherapist before buying essential oils. There may be some that you are sensitive to and he or she can advise you further.

BUYING ESSENTIAL OILS

Essential oils are the diluted essences from fruit, flowers, and trees, and it takes a great deal of work to produce even a tiny amount of essential oil. These oils are therefore expensive, but they are incredibly potent— a little will go a very long way. They are usually sold in ⅓-ounce (10-milliliter) bottles, which contain, on average, about 200 drops. As you can see from the recipes, 200 drops can go a very long way.

Use the following guidelines when buying oils. They will help you to find the best-quality oils and those with the highest therapeutic value.

🌿 Always buy oils in a dark glass bottle. Sunlight is the biggest enemy of essential oils and causes rapid deterioration. Always buy from stores with a high turnover, where the oils are not kept on a shelf exposed to sunlight.

🌿 If you can, buy oils with a dropper insert already in the top of the bottle. This makes it much easier to measure drops correctly. Always practice using the dropper before you make up a recipe—some droppers release the oil at a much faster rate than others.

🌿 Only buy small quantities of essential oils and blend as required with carrier oils.

🌿 Never buy essential oils in plastic containers or decant them into plastic containers afterward. Essential oils and plastic are not compatible. Some of the chemicals in plastics interact with the constituents in essential oils, causing damage to the container or spoiling the oil.

🌿 When buying, look for the phrase "pure essential oil" on the bottle. Only pure, undiluted essential oils can be used effectively in aromatherapy. This applies as much for use in burners and baths as for massage. Any oil you buy that isn't pure essential oil may smell nice, but it won't have the same therapeutic effect as a pure oil. Similarly, don't buy anything labeled "aromatherapy oil."

🌿 Buy the most expensive oils you can. Price is a good indication of quality. If you see a shelf of different oils that are all the same price, don't buy any of them. Neroli, for example, can be twenty times more expensive than lavender. Buy from a reputable source.

STORING ESSENTIAL OILS

All essential oils will deteriorate unless they are stored correctly. If left unopened and stored in perfect condition, they could probably keep for five years or more. Once opened, however, they deteriorate rapidly because air gets inside the bottle. Each time the top is taken off more air travels inside and eventually causes oxidization, which in turn causes the oil to deteriorate. A few simple pointers will help you prolong the life and therapeutic value of your oils so you can get the best out of them down to the last drop.

- Always store bottles of oil in a cool, dark place, away from heat and light, with caps firmly on. Kept this way, oils should have a shelf life of eighteen months. If you live in a hot climate, they can be stored in the refrigerator, taking care to keep them well labeled where children can't reach them. Some oils, such as benzoin, will thicken and solidify when stored in a refrigerator but will soon thin out when removed.

- Some oils, especially the citrus oils, have very poor keeping qualities. Once opened, they may only keep for three or four months. You may notice that they have a slightly fishy smell, in which case do not use. Others such as myrrh and patchouli improve with age.

- Don't allow water to get inside a bottle because it will spoil the oil.

- Carrier oils, such as almond and grapeseed, should be bought fresh regularly and used within three to six months, depending on the oil. They can be kept in the refrigerator to help maintain freshness, but don't use them for massage while still cold!

- Once an essential oil is added to a carrier oil, its shelf life is reduced dramatically—down to just a few months. Make up small quantities of your own oils and aim to use them within three months or so. Wheatgerm oil can be added to a blend to help it keep (it is a natural antioxidant). Jojoba oil also has very good keeping qualities, as well as being highly moisturizing.

HANDLING ESSENTIAL OILS

Always take great care when handling essential oils.

- Keep all essential oils out of the sight and reach of children.

- Do not take essential oils internally.

- Mop up accidental spills—essential oils will leave a mark, especially on polished surfaces.

- When making up oil blends at home, make sure all bottles and utensils are clean and dry. If you are preparing large quantities of oils (unlikely during pregnancy but maybe later if you are making oil blends as presents), make sure the room is well ventilated. Essential oils can be overpowering. Always wear rubber gloves to protect the hands.

🌺 Keep away from the eyes. If you accidentally get essential oil in the eyes, wash them out with plenty of water. Consult a doctor if redness or irritation persists.

🌺 Do not use undiluted essential oils on the skin, apart from lavender and tea tree and then only in very tiny quantities.

🌺 Always consult a qualified aromatherapist before using essential oils if you suffer from allergies or have any medical condition, such as eczema, high blood pressure, or epilepsy, that may be affected by their use.

🌺 If you are pregnant, use only those oils that are recommended for use during pregnancy (see pages 32–36) and never exceed the amount stated in the recipe.

🌺 Always think in drops when using essential oils, and never be tempted to use more drops than instructed.

🌺 Don't self-diagnose. Always consult your doctor about any medical problem. More and more doctors are becoming sympathetic toward complementary medicine and are perfectly happy to let their patients try other therapies. Aromatherapy is a proven way to help your body heal itself, but first you must know what you are trying to heal.

6

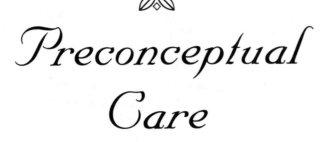

Preconceptual Care

My clients often ask for my feelings about preconceptual care and my reply is always the same—it takes two to make a baby. A prospective mother should only welcome top-quality sperm for top-quality eggs, and time should be spent getting her body as healthy as possible so this can be achieved.

In the real world, some of us won't have the chance to plan a baby. Babies have a habit of arriving at the most unexpected times. But if you are starting with a clean slate, a prebirth plan should start six months before conception. Obviously, the longer you spend on this plan, the better; but if you're in a hurry, then three months will do. Any couple who wishes to plan a baby should individually take responsibility for the care of their own bodies. The general plan involves basic, commonsense guidelines:

- Stop smoking and avoid unnecessary drugs.

- Avoid known pollutants or chemicals.

- Eat a well-balanced and healthy diet (plenty of vegetables, fruits, proteins, and so on), and increase your intake of foods rich in zinc and B vitamins.

- Cut down on stimulants such as tea, coffee, and alcohol (too much alcohol can have an effect on sperm production). Also avoid too much fat or sugar in your diet.

- Watch your weight and exercise to keep your body well toned and supple. Get plenty of rest.

- Stop using oral contraceptives.

- If you have health problems or worries about genetically inherited diseases, see your doctor. If you suffer from minor or stress-related health problems, see an aromatherapist.

FAILURE TO CONCEIVE

Obviously, a couple who tries but consistently fails to conceive should see their doctor. They should continue to follow the general guidelines for preconceptual care in order to prepare their bodies in the event of conception.

Many couples learn that there are no medical reasons for their failure to conceive, yet they still fail to do so. They become increasingly disappointed and experience feelings of guilt, resentment, and tension. Aromatherapy can help with these feelings. Many women I treat may come to me for other reasons, but they eventually mention their anxieties over their failure to conceive.

I do not suggest that the following oils are fertility formulas, but they can greatly reduce the tension between two people who are experiencing these difficult circumstances. Try them along with the general preconceptual care guidelines.

AROMAHELP

Essential Oils

I use the following oils to help people with problems conceiving.

Rose. Known as the perfect skin oil, rose (either *Rosa centiflora* or *Rosa damascena*) is also described as a uterine tonic because it cleanses and regulates the uterus. I find it helpful for clients with premenstrual tension or painful, heavy periods. It is also a good tension reliever and is reputed to have aphrodisiac qualities. Although it is a very feminine oil, rose is thought to increase semen production and is useful in a massage or bath blend for both partners.

Geranium. Geranium is an aromatic oil with many properties. It has a tonic action on the entire body and a hormonal balancing effect on the reproductive system. It is an excellent oil for any condition where anxiety and stress may be a factor . . . and it smells lovely too!

Sandalwood. Sandalwood oil has a heavy, lingering aroma and is highly prized for its effect on male impotence. It is a highly relaxing oil and works well where depression has led to sexual problems or when there is anxiety.

Ylang-Ylang. An exotically scented oil frequently used in relaxing massage and bath blends, ylang-ylang gives a pleasantly romantic smell to the skin. It is used in cases of nervous tension, anxiety, and impotence.

Massage Oils

Use the following oils for a relaxing massage. Pay special attention to the lower back, abdomen, groin, and hip area. Don't use the oils directly on the delicate genital area because they could sting.

Massage Oil for Her. Add 15 drops of geranium oil and 5 drops of rose oil to 2½ tablespoons (50 milliliters) of almond oil. Mix well.

Massage Oil for Him. Add 5 drops of clary sage oil, 5 drops of rose oil, 5 drops of geranium oil, and 5 drops of either sandalwood or ylang-ylang oil to 2½ tablespoons (50 milliliters) of almond oil. Mix well.

Bath Mixes

Try the following bath mixes. These baths can be enjoyed up to four times a week. Aim to have at least two baths and two massages each per week while on this program.

Blend 1. Blend 1 is relaxing and can be used by both of you during the evening. To a warm bath, add 4 drops of geranium oil, 2 drops of rose oil, and 2 drops of clary sage oil. Swish the water to disperse the oil. Relax and soak for ten to fifteen minutes.

Blend 2. Blend 2 is for women to use as a morning bath. Add 4 drops of geranium oil and 2 drops of rose oil to a full bath. Swish the water to disperse the oil. Soak for ten minutes.

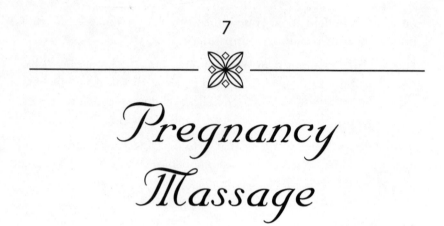

7

Pregnancy Massage

Pregnancy is one time in a woman's life when she needn't feel guilty about occasionally indulging herself. There's no greater treat than a body massage to uplift the spirits.

Regular aromatherapy body massages throughout pregnancy—coupled with regular visits to the prenatal clinic—are sure ways of helping a mother-to-be look and feel her best. An aromatherapy massage can help relax the entire body and relieve the feelings of fatigue so common in the early and later stages of pregnancy. A massage is sheer bliss for aching sides, back, and legs. The whole body is toned, posture is improved, and stiffness that comes with the heaviness of pregnancy is alleviated. Massage can help the circulation, lower high blood pressure, and improve the complexion, as well as keep the skin nourished, supple, and elastic, which helps prevent stretch marks. Toward the last month of pregnancy a woman can often feel physically and sexually unattractive, even if other people don't see her that way. An aromatherapy massage can help the mother-to-be feel good about herself and keep her confidence in her looks.

A PROFESSIONAL MASSAGE

During pregnancy and postpartum, clients consult me because an aromatherapy massage makes them feel good, for treatment of a minor problem, or for a variety of other reasons. Most pregnant clients book their first massage after they have had their first prenatal appointment, usually at around twelve weeks. I only recommend an aromatherapy treatment after that time.

I believe in working in total cooperation with the client's doctor, midwife, or other caregiver. By doing so, she can feel secure in the knowledge that we are working as a team for her benefit, making her pregnancy experience a very special one.

Each client is treated as an individual. Two people who visit me may have the same complaint, but they might require different approaches to treatment and entirely different oils. To help me determine a client's needs, I like to give a thirty-minute consultation before I begin treatment. Some of the things I ask about are diet and exercise, relevant medical history, the client's general health, a history of previous pregnancies, and allergies she may have (in case she may be allergic to any of the oils). I also must determine if there are medical reasons why it may be inadvisable for the client to have a massage, such as a threatened miscarriage or a present illness, and I take note of special concerns such as back problems or varicose veins.

After the initial consultation I advise the client about the appropriate form of treatment, perhaps a course of aromatherapy treatments with oils to use at home. I always make the oil blends to suit the individual, and I usually ask her to keep them on for six to eight hours after a massage for maximum absorption. It is quite normal after a first aromatherapy treatment to have a reaction—the client may feel slightly tired, she may feel as if she is coming down with the flu, or she may have a slight headache. These reactions are signs that the body is throwing out toxins. On the day of an aromatherapy massage it is best for the client to take it easy after the treatment in order to allow the full benefit of aromatherapy to work. The next day she should feel relaxed and rested. Having said this, I have never treated a mother-to-be who has experienced any side effects after a treatment. Those who sometimes have side effects are those I treat for conditions such as cellulite, arthritis, stress, or conditions where there are toxins to eliminate and where strong oils are used. Clients should avoid having a large meal just before or just after an aromatherapy treatment and should drink plenty of water to help flush out toxins.

When I first see a pregnant woman in my aromatherapy clinic, I usually begin with a back massage. I ask my client to sit on the massage bed wrapped in towels, with her feet resting on a stool. A towel-covered pillow is placed underneath the stomach for total support. The back takes so much strain during pregnancy that quite often my clients purr with relief when it is massaged.

I then ask the mother-to-be to lie down and support her with as many pillows as necessary to make her comfortable. Some women need to be practically sitting up because they find they can't breathe properly lying down; most need pillows for support behind the knees and in the small of the back where many women develop a hollow during pregnancy, I then massage the legs, feet, and ankles, which encourages unwanted fluid to drain (it is very common to have fluid retention in the lower body during pregnancy). I then oil and stroke the abdomen, using very gentle movements without applying pressure. This helps keep the skin supple and elastic and relieves tension at the sides of the body and the diaphragm. At all times I respect that I am actually massaging two people, and it's lovely to feel the baby move as I stroke the oils over the mother's abdomen. I am sure some babies kick and nudge their mothers when I stop because they want me to continue.

After the abdomen has been massaged, the pregnant woman can change her position if she wants to. I finish with a face, neck, shoulder, and head massage—unless the client dislikes oil on her hair or is going out after treatment. The oil for the face massage is individually tailored to suit the condition of the client's skin.

By the time the massage is over, the mother-to-be is totally relaxed and may even be asleep. I allow her to rest for a while before she leaves my treatment room feeling refreshed and content or, as one mother put it, "completely at peace with the world." All pregnant clients whom I treat report that they sleep like proverbial logs after treatment, and they find it much easier to relax at prenatal classes.

GIVING A MASSAGE AT HOME

Naturally, the best person to give an aromatherapy massage is a qualified practitioner. But it is possible to have a massage at home with a willing partner. Many fathers-to-be feel a very special prebirth bond with the baby by gently massaging their partner's abdomen—they feel the baby move under their hands. Massage is also a valuable way of bringing a couple closer together, especially during the later stages of pregnancy when a woman often feels unattractive and feels her husband is not sexually interested in her. In turn, the husband can feel threatened by his partner's total absorption in the baby and may worry that making love could harm the child. A couple can touch and remain close through a massage.

Try to get your partner to massage you regularly during pregnancy, especially if he is going to be with you during labor. Have a well-practiced set of movements planned—it's no use if he finds out you hate having your feet rubbed when you get into the labor room. He should know well in advance what you like and what is soothing so he won't need to be instructed when it's really important. Remind him that tempers often get frayed during labor, especially at the end of the first stage, and you may not feel like talking to him.

Many men are not used to giving a massage, so it may be worth giving him a foot or back massage so he can feel the variations in pressure. It is especially useful for your partner or other labor coach to have a prelabor massage if he or she is going to be present at the birth, if only so that he or she can experience how annoying it is to have a poor massage and how important it is to know which movements are preferred.

TIPS FOR HOME MASSAGE

Here are a few tips for the person who is going to massage a mother-to-be:

- Collect everything you will need—such as massage oil, extra towels, and so forth—before you start.

- Make the atmosphere as calm and relaxed as possible. Make sure the room is warm, dim the lights if necessary, and perhaps play some soothing music. I don't advise scenting the room with essential oils, purely because, if you are using them in a massage oil, their aroma will naturally perfume the air.

- Don't do it in a hurry. If you haven't much time, just massage part of the body, say the back. If the pregnant woman is particularly exhausted, the best massage is a leg and foot one. You may well find she drops off to sleep halfway through.

🌱 After three months of pregnancy, don't allow the woman to lie on her stomach.

🌱 The ideal position for a back massage for the mother-to-be is to sit astride a chair supported by cushions. The rest of the massage can be done on a bed covered with towels, with plenty of cushions behind the back so that she is almost sitting. As pregnancy advances, get her to lie supported by as many cushions as are comfortable for her. She may find it easier with pillows or cushions under her knees.

🌱 When giving a whole-body massage, cover her with towels and only expose the part of the body that is actually being massaged. The body temperature lowers when lying still, so she can get cold.

🌱 Keep all movements gentle. Don't worry about being a practiced massage therapist. Just use gentle movement that is relaxing and feels right. Encourage her to let you know what feels good.

🌱 Massage those areas where there is tension, and always massage toward the heart.

🌱 Don't press on varicose veins; just glide gently around them.

🌱 Don't massage the mother-to-be immediately after she has had a hot bath. Although a massage feels wonderful on warm, relaxed muscles, skin that is still perspiring can't absorb oils well. It is better to allow her to cool down a little before you begin.

- Avoid the lower abdomen and back during the first three months of pregnancy. During the rest of pregnancy, avoid deep pressure on the abdomen and lower back.

- Don't massage if the mother-to-be feels unwell or has any bleeding (in which case she should consult her midwife or doctor). Never massage anyone with a fever.

- The order in which you massage different parts of the body doesn't matter (see pages 48–50 for the way in which I give a professional massage), but if you are giving a full-body massage, it might be easier to do the back first with the pregnant woman sitting astride a chair.

- As a rough guide, allow about ten minutes for a foot and leg massage, ten minutes for a back massage, and five minutes or less for the abdomen.

PREPARING A MASSAGE OIL

The following recipe makes an ideal oil for massage during pregnancy.

Standard Pregnancy Massage Oil

Make a base oil by mixing 4 tablespoons (80 milliliters) of sweet almond oil with 1 tablespoon (20 milliliters) of avocado oil. Add 10 drops of tangerine oil and 5 drops of neroli oil or 10 drops of tangerine oil and 5 drops of lavender oil.

BACK AND SHOULDER MASSAGE

The woman can either lie on her side near enough to the edge of the bed for you to massage her comfortably, or, for better access and results, she can sit astride a chair supported by cushions. With gentle, upward strokes using the standard pregnancy massage oil (above), glide the hands straight up either side of the spine and up over the shoulder blades, smoothing them down the side of the body and molding them to the shape. At the waist area, gently massage in circular movements to relieve the tension from overstretched ligaments. Always be very gentle in later pregnancy when massaging the lower back.

BODY MASSAGE

With the mother-to-be comfortably settled and supported on towels and pillows, stroke the oil in delicate, clockwise movements around the abdomen. Remember, you are massaging two people (you may well be reminded of this if the baby gives a quick kick). Glide your hands to either side of the waist—or what was once the waist—and gently up and down the sides of the body. This relieves the stretching and pulling so often felt there during pregnancy.

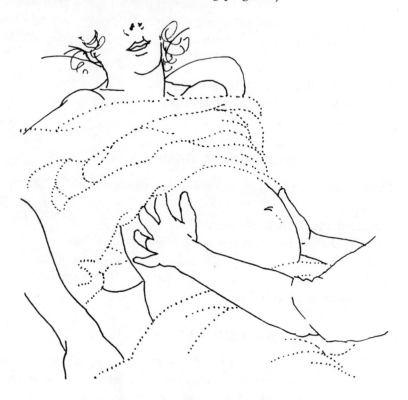

FOOT AND LEG MASSAGE

This is a particularly good remedy for insomnia and helps relieve fluid retention. Use either the standard pregnancy massage oil (see page 53) or, if the woman is having problems with aching feet and legs, you may want to use the soothing leg and foot oil (see page 61). The mother-to-be can sit whichever way she feels comfortable, or she can lie down propped up on pillows with towels under her feet. Make gentle upward strokes, gliding the hands from ankles to thighs and back to the ankles again, but don't put any pressure on the downward slide. Then sweep under the foot and gently up the legs again. Try to get into a rhythm.

Rotate the ankles first one way and then the other. It also helps to flex the foot a few times. These actions bring a lot of relief to heavy legs. Massage the oil all over the feet and around the ankles. With hands cupped around one foot and fingers steadying the front of the foot, use the thumbs to make circular pressures on the sole. Gently squeeze and press the foot as though you were trying to make it into a pliable piece of dough.

AFTER YOU HAVE BEEN MASSAGED

Relax and enjoy the feeling of being pampered. It is best to leave the oils on to allow them to soak into the body and work properly. It can take anywhere from twenty minutes to seven hours for oils to work their way fully into the body via the skin, but they will be thoroughly absorbed by then so the skin won't be left feeling greasy. It is best to have a massage just before bed, allowing the oils to soak in overnight and then bathing in the morning. The skin will feel soft, glowing, and wonderful.

MASSAGING YOUR BABY

Don't forget when you are applying anti-stretch-mark oils on the stomach to gently feel the form of your baby. I encourage all my clients and their partners to talk to their unborn babies. The best time to do this is during the daily "oiling session," when they can gently stroke him or her. If the baby is very active at night, try giving a prebirth massage then.

It is generally thought that in the first few weeks after birth babies will respond to touch when they are upset, because they are used to their mother's touch. Several of my clients who had not used aromatherapy massage with previous pregnancies were convinced that after birth, their "aroma" babies responded far more quickly to being comforted.

8

Aromahelp for Discomforts During Pregnancy

Don't think that you will get all—or even any—of the discomforts discussed below. Pregnancies vary from woman to woman, and even from baby to baby, but being prepared for the discomforts is half the battle. If you have symptoms you are particularly worried about, consult your doctor or midwife at your regular prenatal checkups.

BACK, WAIST, AND GROIN ACHE

As pregnancy progresses, the extra weight around the stomach pulls at the ligaments around the waist and spine. During the last three months, hormonal changes make the supporting joints and ligaments relax and prepare for labor. It is then that backache—especially in the lower back—is a problem. The added weight results in a change in posture that can bring about aches in the groin area.

I generally advise women during pregnancy to do the following:

🍃 Take it easy. If you are aching all over, it is usually a sign you are overdoing things, so slow down.

🍃 Take care with posture. The natural impulse as you get larger is to stick the stomach out, but try to keep the back straight instead of curved. Take care not to overstrain when bending and lifting and use your legs more than your back.

AROMAHELP

🍃 A regular weekly aromatherapy massage from a friend or partner is beneficial for strain and backache (see chapter 6). Use the standard pregnancy massage oil found on page 53.

🍃 Try a relaxing warm bath at the end of the day. Add 2 drops of lavender oil to the bathwater.

COMPULSORY BEDREST

A threatened miscarriage, high blood pressure, or multiple pregnancy means that some women must spend much more time inactive than they'd really like to. If you are unlucky enough to have to spend some or all of your pregnancy resting in bed, the most important thing is to calm down and take it easy.

AROMAHELP

🍃 A massage with essential oils will help you relax. A full-body massage may not be possible, but get a partner or friend to give you hand, foot, or facial massages.

🍃 Don't forget to oil your stomach, breasts, and thighs to help keep the skin supple.

🍃 For a relaxing atmosphere in your room, add 2 drops of any of the following essential oils to hot water in a burner or lightbulb ring: geranium, lavender, lemon, bergamot, or ylang-ylang. The vapors will fill the room.

CYSTITIS

Cystitis is a painful inflammation of the bladder and lower urinary passages that can occur more frequently during pregnancy as the growing uterus presses on the bladder. It can also signify a bacterial infection. Mild symptoms include an uncomfortable feeling in the bladder and the need to urinate frequently. More severe symptoms include burning, painful urination with fever, abdominal pain, and back pain. Some women describe the sensation as "trying to urinate through cut glass"; others compare it to a nagging itch they can't reach. The symptoms may intensify when the woman is lying down, so it's best to walk around the room and keep active. If cystitis is accompanied by a fever or severe pain, or if symptoms persist, see a doctor immediately. It could be an indication of a kidney infection.

You can help prevent an attack of cystitis by following the advice given below:

❧ Flush out the bladder by drinking plenty of water or lemon barley water. Current research also suggests that cranberry juice is helpful. The more you drink, the more comfortable the bladder becomes and the easier it is to urinate. Never go for too long without emptying the bladder.

❧ When you feel you may be getting cystitis try to keep warm, particularly from the waist down. If you have an attack at night, a hot water bottle placed between the top of the legs can be comforting.

❧ Make sure the genital area is washed every day with mild soap and water and rinsed well. Cystitis can be brought on by infection, so when on the toilet, wipe your bottom from front to back to prevent infection from the bowel finding its way into the bladder.

❧ To avoid "honeymoon" cystitis, brought on by intercourse and local irritation of the urethra, make sure that after making love you empty the bladder and wash the genital area.

❧ If you are a frequent cystitis sufferer, avoid the food or drink you know can bring on an attack—usually alcohol or spicy foods. One client of mine gets cystitis every time she drinks more than one glass of red wine.

✢ Take a warm sitz bath, to which you have added either 2 drops of lavender oil, 2 drops of sandalwood oil, 2 drops of bergamot oil, or 2 drops of chamomile oil. Mix the oil well into the water. Soak for five to ten minutes.

✢ Or have a full bath. To the warm bathwater (never too hot), add either 2 drops of lavender oil, 2 drops of sandalwood oil, or 1 drop of bergamot oil and 1 drop of sandalwood oil. Swish the water around to disperse the oil. Then relax and soak for ten to fifteen minutes in the warm water.

Take a bath with the oils mentioned above whenever you have an attack of cystitis. You may get the desire to urinate in the bath, because the warm water will ease the burning and discomfort. Don't worry if you do. I've heard doctors advise their patients to do this many times, so think of it as "doctor's orders."

FATIGUE

Fatigue is a natural part of pregnancy. You must expect to feel tired, particularly toward the end of your pregnancy when the extra weight and demands the baby is making on your body all conspire to slow you down.

Listen to your body. If you feel sleepy, take a nap during the day and don't feel guilty. Put your feet up whenever you can and accept all offers from friends or relatives to help with the shopping, cleaning, or other chores. Make the most of it while you can.

AROMAHELP

When you need to unwind during the day or night, slip into a comfortable bath with essential oils. Depending on which aroma you prefer, add either of the following combinations: 2 drops of lavender oil, 1 drop of mandarin oil, and 1 drop of ylang-ylang oil; or 1 drop of lavender oil, 1 drop of mandarin oil, and 2 drops of ylang-ylang oil. Soak in the bath for ten to fifteen minutes.

FEELING FAINT

Feeling faint happens quite often during pregnancy because the blood pressure is low. If you feel faint, sit down and put your feet up.

AROMAHELP

Try this simple inhalation. Place 1 drop of geranium oil on a tissue or clean handkerchief. Sit back, relax, and sniff as required.

FLUID RETENTION

Fluid retention is very common in later pregnancy. The first sign is usually that the rings on your fingers become tight. Your ankles and feet may swell, making your shoes feel cramped at the end of the day, and you may feel very tired. Heat can aggravate fluid retention, making it more of a problem during a summer pregnancy.

If you are retaining fluids, try the following:

❧ Rest with your feet up—preferably higher than your head—as often as possible to allow the fluid to drain away from the ankles and feet. Avoid standing still or being on your feet for long periods of time, and take breaks to move around when you are on long car journeys.

❧ Watch your diet. Salt and sugar both aggravate fluid retention, so check the contents of preprepared meals—they often have a high salt content. Cut down on tea and coffee.

If fluid retention is still a problem after a few simple measures, then see your doctor or midwife for a blood pressure check and urinalysis. Don't take any diuretic pills unless they are prescribed by your doctor.

AROMAHELP

❧ A foot and leg massage can help, by pushing the fluid up and removing it as well as by relieving discomfort. Massage the legs and feet with the soothing leg and foot oil (below). You can either do this yourself or get someone to do it for you. Starting at the ankle, massage with firm upward strokes over the knee to the upper thigh (or just massage the lower leg to the knee). Glide hands down and repeat. Rotate the ankles first one way and then the other. It also helps to flex the foot a few times—this brings relief to heavy legs. Massage the feet by pressing and rubbing them. Make circular pressures with thumbs over the soles. Stroke the front of the feet firmly down from the base of the toes to the ankles and circle around the ankles.

🦋 Footbaths can also help. For a soothing footbath, add 1 drop of geranium oil and 1 drop of lemon oil to a bowl of coolish water. Soak your feet in this mixture for as long as needed.

Soothing Leg and Foot Oil
To 1½ tablespoons (30 milliliters) of almond oil or unperfumed gel (ask your pharmacist if unsure), add 2 drops of lavender oil and 2 drops of geranium oil.

HEMORRHOIDS

Hemorrhoids are congested veins around the rectum and anal canal. They can be itchy and sore and can make opening the bowels very painful; they can even bleed. Hemorrhoids are aggravated by the pelvic congestion that results from pregnancy.

Avoid getting constipated—eat a high-fiber diet with lots of fruit and vegetables and drink plenty of water. If you are constipated, don't strain when on the toilet. Straining will make the hemorrhoids worse. According to medical opinion, sitting on the toilet for too long actually encourages hemorrhoids. You may find it more comfortable to wipe your bottom with a damp cotton washcloth after opening the bowels.

AROMAHELP

🦋 Take a warm (not hot) sitz bath to which you have added 2 drops of geranium oil and 2 drops of cypress oil. Soak in it for ten minutes.

🦋 Or soak a cloth or a cotton pad in the same solution and hold it against the back passage. You may find this easier to do while sitting on the toilet.

🦋 Try a compress. Using a compress may sound like torture, but it brings wonderful relief. To a small bowl of water, add 2 drops of geranium oil and 2 drops of cypress oil. Soak a cloth in this mixture, then wrap the cloth around a small bag of ice cubes. Hold it against the anus for one minute (or slightly longer if you really need to). Repeat every four hours and after opening the bowels.

🌿 Apply a small amount—about a teaspoonful—of the hemorrhoid gel (below) to the hemorrhoids after opening the bowels and whenever they are sore and itchy.

Hemorrhoid Gel

To 2½ tablespoons (50 milliliters) of aloe gel or any lubricating gel, add 5 drops of cypress oil and 5 drops of geranium oil. Mix well.

INDIGESTION AND HEARTBURN

Indigestion can occur throughout pregnancy. Heartburn is a burning sensation in the lower part of the chest that is sometimes accompanied by small amounts of regurgitated acidic fluid. Heartburn is more common toward the end of pregnancy.

The following tips should help prevent attacks of indigestion and heartburn:

🌿 Look at your diet and avoid the foods that cause indigestion or heartburn, usually spicy, fried, or dairy foods. Don't overeat.

🌿 Toward the end of the pregnancy, as the baby gets larger, the stomach may be rather squashed, so it may be better to eat small meals more frequently.

🌿 If indigestion or heartburn is an intense problem, you may think about food combining (that is, avoiding mixing foods that fight, such as protein and starch) to help digestion. There are several books available on this subject.

AROMAHELP

Use the standard pregnancy massage oil (see page 53) to gently massage the solar plexus between the breasts and abdomen. Or use the indigestion massage oil (below).

Indigestion Massage Oil

To ½ tablespoon (10 milliliters) of any carrier oil, add either 2 drops of sandalwood oil, 2 drops of orange oil, or 2 drops of mandarin oil. Mix well.

Sandalwood oil would be the best choice of essential oil if you have it. It makes an excellent massage oil to use anytime you have indigestion.

INSOMNIA

Toward the end of pregnancy, and especially in the last month, many women find it increasingly difficult to sleep, particularly if the baby is active and kicking at night. Try resting the stomach on a pillow to make lying on your side more comfortable. It can also help if you increase the number of pillows you sleep on from two to four to help your breathing. Also, wear loose nightclothes and cut out tea and coffee in the evening. A warm milky drink can help the last thing at night.

AROMAHELP

❧ A gentle massage before going to bed is one way to relax and sleep well. If there is no time for a full-body massage, ask a friend or partner to give you a soporific foot massage. Use the standard pregnancy massage oil (see page 53).

❧ A relaxing bath just before bed can help. To a warm bath, add 3 drops of lavender, mandarin, or ylang-ylang oil. Swish the water to disperse the oil. Relax and soak for ten minutes.

❧ Scent the bedroom to induce sleep. To a burner, diffuser, or bowl of hot water, add 2–3 drops of lavender or ylang-ylang oil or a mixture of these two oils.

LEG CRAMPS

Leg cramps are very painful, shooting muscle spasms. They are common in pregnancy—especially, it seems, in the middle of the night—but no one really knows why. Calcium is supposed to help, so eat plenty of calcium-rich foods. During a cramp attack, don't stretch the leg out with the toes pointed. Instead, rub the calf and pull the foot up toward you; then hang on to the foot until the pain passes (as your pregnancy progresses, you will have to do this sitting down with your legs bent).

AROMAHELP

Massage will help. Try the leg cramp massage oil (below). If you have leg cramps most evenings or nights, use ¼ tablespoon (5 milliliters) of the oil every night for a week and repeat as you need to.

Leg Cramp Massage Oil

To 1½ tablespoons (30 milliliters) of almond oil, add 2 drops of lavender and 2 drops of geranium oil. Mix well.

MORNING SICKNESS

Morning sickness is often one of the first symptoms of pregnancy. The awful feeling of nausea that comes with morning sickness, contrary to the name, can happen at any time of the day, though it is more common first thing in the morning. It can also continue well past the first three months of pregnancy.

The sense of smell becomes more acute during pregnancy. Some women find they can't tolerate even normal household smells or smells they usually enjoy, such as their favorite perfume. For this reason, it's difficult to recommend an essential oil for morning sickness. There is little that aromatherapy can do to help, but try the following general tips:

* Most important, avoid all food or smells that make you feel queasy. The usual culprits are coffee, dairy foods, cigarette smoke, and fried food. If cooking makes you feel sick, then get someone else to cook for a while.

* Avoid getting out of bed too quickly in the morning. Sit up slowly and keep still for about ten minutes. Try to take things much more slowly during the day—rushing about can bring on nausea.

* Upon waking, sip Indian or China tea very slowly. If no one is on hand to wait on you, keep a thermos flask on your night table (with some powdered milk if you drink your tea light). Alternatively, try

sipping hot water with the juice of half a lemon; or infuse a small piece of fresh gingerroot in a cup of boiling hot water (remove the ginger after five minutes and drink slowly); or add a pinch of dried ginger to a cup of hot water (do not use essential oil of ginger).

🌿 When you wake, nibble on some dry toast, plain dry crackers, or thin slices of crispy apple to help settle the stomach.

🌿 Don't take over-the-counter medications unless your doctor has approved them. If your vomiting is severe, see your doctor or midwife.

AROMAHELP

It is difficult to prescribe an essential oil for morning sickness, but some women find that 1–2 drops of lemon oil in a burner or diffuser in the bedroom will help relieve nausea. Use whenever you feel nauseous. If the feeling of sickness persists throughout the day, try the same remedy in whatever room you happen to be in.

NOSEBLEEDS AND CONGESTION

Nosebleeds and nasal congestion are common side effects of pregnancy as a result of increased blood supply to the nasal passages. Both usually end as soon as pregnancy is over, but nosebleeds can be a sign of high blood pressure, so inform your doctor or midwife at your next prenatal checkup.

AROMAHELP

🌿 An inhalation will remove the pressure on the nasal passages if you have a stuffy nose, but never use this treatment if you have a nosebleed because it will make it worse. To a bowl of hot water, add 2 drops of eucalyptus or tea tree oil and inhale the steam for a couple of minutes.

🌿 A facial massage can also help deal with congestion. To ½ table-spoon (10 milliliters) of jojoba or grapeseed oil, add 1 drop of lavender oil to make a massage oil. Using this massage oil on the fingertips, press and release the fingers gently along the cheekbones to loosen any congestion.

If you have a nosebleed, pinch the bottom of the nostrils quite hard for a short while—a minute or two—and it should stop. Or use the compress below. Obviously, if you have frequent or severe nosebleeds, consult your doctor or midwife.

Compress for Nosebleeds

Place about 8 ounces (240 milliliters) of very cold water in a bowl (add ice if necessary). Add 1 drop of cypress oil or 1 drop of lemon oil.

Agitate the water, soak a clean cloth in it, squeeze, then use the cloth as a compress by laying it on top of the nose for a few minutes. The nosebleed should stop.

PALPITATIONS

Palpitations, medically defined as "being aware of the heartbeat," feel like fluttering sensations in the chest; sometimes it feels as though the heart has missed a beat. Palpitations can be caused by too much caffeine or by stress. Those who are nervous are particularly prone to palpitations, which are often wrongly described as a rapid heartbeat (tachycardia). However, because a rapid heartbeat can also be caused by stress and fear, the same essential oils can help both conditions.

If you suffer from palpitations, cut down on all stimulants, such as tea, coffee, and soft drinks. See your doctor or midwife if the palpitations are severe.

AROMAHELP

- To ½ tablespoon (10 milliliters) of a carrier oil, add 1 drop of neroli oil or 1 drop of ylang-ylang oil. Massage this into either the feet, the back of the hands, or the abdomen.

- Ylang-ylang oil can also be used in a diffuser, burner, or bowl of hot water to scent the room and to encourage a calming effect.

PREPARING THE PERINEAL AREA

The perineum is the skin between the vagina and the anus. It will be stretched during labor, so it needs to be given a little help beforehand. The perineum is a very sensitive area so you should never apply essential oils to it. During the last eight weeks of your pregnancy, gently rub it daily with ¼ teaspoonful of jojoba oil. Jojoba is highly lubricating. It will help the skin become more supple and may prevent tearing during delivery.

SKIN, HAIR, AND NAIL PROBLEMS

The skin during pregnancy varies from woman to woman. Some find that their skin, hair, and nails have never looked better and they truly "bloom"; others suffer from greasy skin and lank hair.

If pregnancy is taking its toll on your skin, take the normal precautions: make sure you have a good diet (with plenty of vitamin C) and try to get as much sleep as you can.

Getting a professional pedicure or manicure to keep the nails looking good can really boost morale during pregnancy. Always keep your hair well washed, either by yourself or by a friend if it gets difficult to bend over a basin in the later stages of pregnancy.

Many pregnant women tell me they are often hot and their skin can get quite clammy. An atomizer filled with orange flower water can be used to spray on the face. It can also be helpful to use when you are in labor.

AROMAHELP

Your aromatherapist can advise you about skin and hair care, depending on your individual needs, but the facial massage oil (below) can also help. Lightly massage this oil into the face about three times a week after cleansing. You will probably find that the oil sinks in completely, but if there is any excess, blot it off with a tissue. Never go to bed with an oily face because it could cause puffiness under the eyes in the morning.

See chapter 12 for more recipes for skin care.

Facial Massage Oil
To ½ tablespoon (10 milliliters) of jojoba oil, add 1–2 drops of lavender, neroli, or sandalwood oil.

SORE BREASTS

One of the first signs of pregnancy is sore or swollen breasts that feel much like premenstrual breasts do. It is important to wear a well-fitting bra throughout pregnancy to give your breasts proper support. You may have to change sizes several times as they gradually swell. Have your breasts measured if you are in doubt as to their size. You can do this in any lingerie department of a large store. If your breasts feel very heavy and uncomfortable, wear a bra—preferably a cotton one—at night.

AROMAHELP

- Use the anti-stretch-mark oil (see page 69) to massage the breasts. Regular use will help avoid stretch marks.

- Bathe regularly in warm water to which you have added 2 drops of lavender oil or 2 drops of geranium oil. Lie back and let the water cover your breasts; or soak a washcloth in the water and hold it to your breasts.

- Try this compress: To 8 ounces (240 milliliters) of water (it can be either hot or cold, whichever gives the most relief), add 2 drops of lavender oil and 2 drops of geranium oil. Soak a cloth in the water, and then hold the cloth to your breasts.

SORE OR BLEEDING GUMS

Soft and bleeding gums are more common during pregnancy because of hormonal changes. They can also be a sign of gum disease, so visit the dentist for a checkup and the hygienist to have your teeth and gums thoroughly cleaned.

Keep your teeth scrupulously clean and floss well between them each time you brush. Make sure you have a good intake of vitamin C.

AROMAHELP

Unfortunately, the essential oils I would normally recommend to treat sore or bleeding gums, such as clove and myrrh, are unsuitable to use during pregnancy. It may help to squeeze some lemon juice in a small glass of water and use as a mouthwash.

STRETCH MARKS

Stretch marks are the thin red streaks that can form on the abdomen, thighs, breasts, hips, buttocks, and tops of the arms during pregnancy. In severe cases stretch marks may bleed. They are the result of a weakening or breakdown of the underlying fibers in the skin. Once these fibers have been overstretched, they will not return to normal after the weight decreases, but the marks will fade from red to silver feathery lines. Women with delicate, fair skin are the most vulnerable. Try to avoid putting on weight too rapidly in pregnancy. A slow gain will allow the skin time to adjust.

AROMAHELP

Aromatherapy encourages the attitude that prevention is better than cure. Tangerine, neroli, and lavender oils have been shown to promote healthy skin cells when combined in either a moisturizing cream or a massage oil. Use the recipe below, or you can use the standard pregnancy massage oil (see page 53) to help to keep the skin supple and elastic and prevent stretch marks.

Apply a small amount of the oil daily and gently massage it into the hips, stomach, thighs, and breasts, paying attention to any area that feels particularly taut or to previous scar tissue. The anti-stretch-mark oil can also help relieve the tightness and itching that come with rapid weight gain, as in a multiple pregnancy.

After the birth, continue using the anti-stretch-mark oil until your weight and figure get back to normal. Surprisingly, stretch marks can occur when weight is decreasing.

Anti-Stretch-Mark Oil

To 4 tablespoons (80 milliliters) of almond oil and 1 tablespoon (20 milliliters) of avocado oil, add either 7 drops of lavender and 5 drops of neroli oil, or 7 drops of lavender and 5 drops of mandarin or tangerine oil, or 5 drops of neroli oil and 7 drops of mandarin or tangerine oil.

VARICOSE VEINS

Varicose veins are purplish dilated veins that often develop in the legs, calves, and even the groin in later pregnancy. They are caused by increased weight, which hinders the return of blood to the legs and can result in throbbing pains and aching legs.

If you had varicose veins before becoming pregnant, they may be more pronounced now, as increased weight causes pressure in the pelvic area. The good news is that if they were brought on by pregnancy, they often disappear fairly quickly afterward.

The following tips should help:

🌿 Avoid standing still or sitting with your legs crossed, which will aggravate varicose veins. A gentle daily walk will help the circulation, as will putting your feet up when you sit. Try to rest with your feet higher than your head as often as possible, and if you have very bad veins and extreme fluid retention, it might be a good idea to slightly raise the end of your bed by placing it on blocks.

🌿 Exercise the calf muscles by flexing the feet up and down. Give the legs a good stretch by rotating the ankles, first one way and then the other.

AROMAHELP

🌿 A warm bath will help relieve throbbing pain (never use hot water because it will aggravate varicose veins). Add 4 drops of lavender oil to the bathwater and swish to disperse. Relax and soak for ten to fifteen minutes.

🌿 Whenever your legs ache, gently stroke the varicose vein leg lotion (below) up them. Never massage below the varicose veins—just glide around the side of them. You could also ask your partner to rub your feet with this wonderfully cooling lotion, stretching and rotating them to aid the circulation.

Varicose Vein Leg Lotion

To 2 ounces (approximately 100 milliliters) of unperfumed lotion, add 5 drops of lemon oil, 5 drops of geranium oil, and 5 drops of cypress oil. Mix well and keep the bottle in the fridge.

YEAST INFECTIONS

A multitude of bacteria live naturally in our intestines. Some of them are highly beneficial to our well-being. If some of these "good" bacteria are destroyed, then the body goes into an unbalanced state and other organisms that also normally live harmlessly in the body can begin to grow and cause infection.

One such organism, a yeastlike fungus called *Candida albicans,* is responsible for an infection of the mucus membranes called a yeast infection or thrush (if in the mouth). Yeast infections can affect the mouth, skin, vagina, and bowel. They can take hold in the vagina when the vaginal tract becomes too alkaline (it needs to be slightly acidic, just like the surface of our skin).

Yeast infections can occur for a variety of reasons. They may occur during or follow a course of antibiotics. Antibiotics attack unwanted bacterial infection, but they also kill off the "good" bacteria that help maintain the acid–alkali balance in the vaginal area. Hormonal changes during pregnancy and postpartum can also upset the acid–alkali balance in the vaginal tract and increase the chances of getting an infection, as can menopause and taking the contraceptive pill. Yeast infections can occur in people with poor health, whose immune systems are worn down, and in those suffering from gross fatigue and stress.

The first sign of a yeast infection is an irritating thick, white discharge rather like cottage cheese. The vaginal tract can become red and sore, and it may bleed a little when touched. There may also be some pain when urinating and during intercourse.

The following advice should help:

🌿 Pay attention to your diet. Cut back on foods that encourage yeast growth—sugar, alcohol, and refined foods. Cut down on tea and coffee; it may also be wise to cut down on fruit. Eat plenty of live natural yogurt containing lactobacillus to redress the balance of friendly bacteria in the intestines. Eat foods rich in B vitamins, such as fresh vegetables and whole-grain cereals.

🌿 Wear cotton underwear and stockings instead of nylons—yeast thrives in damp, unventilated areas.

🌿 Towels and washcloths spread germs. During a yeast infection, don't share bath towels with anyone else, change the towel you use every day, and don't use a washcloth.

🌿 See your doctor if an attack is severe. You may be given vaginal suppositories. Essential oil treatments can be used at the same time as these suppositories.

To prevent further attacks or reinfection, use a condom during intercourse with your partner. Make sure the condoms are well lubricated. If they are too dry, the irritation will make the infection even worse. It is also wise to encourage your partner to obtain treatment at the same time you do. He can use any of the recipes below.

AROMAHELP

Some essential oils, particularly tea tree and lavender, have been shown to inhibit the growth of thrush and other fungal infections. When used in a diluted solution, they can bring relief by alleviating the itching and inflammation, soothing the infected areas, and helping to treat the condition.

 Add 2–4 drops of the yeast essential oil mix (see page 73) to a warm bath. Soak in the water for ten minutes. You can also add 2–3 drops of this mixture to a basin or bidet of warm water and use it to wash the vaginal area. Never use commercial bubble baths if you have a yeast infection. They are too alkaline and can irritate the vagina.

 Use the gentle yeast infection cream (see page 73) to soothe the delicate vulva. Apply three to four times a day.

 In addition to eating live natural yogurt to help restore the "friendly" bacteria in the intestines, many women find that inserting a yogurt and tea tree oil mixture into the vagina not only soothes and stops the intense itch but can prevent full-blown attack from developing. The yogurt and tea tree oil mixture is inserted into the vagina on a tampon, so this method should *never* be used during pregnancy. Only use the tampon method postpartum, when you have been told by your doctor or midwife that you may resume wearing tampons again (see caution below).

Remove enough yogurt from a pot of plain, live yogurt to completely coat a slightly damp tampon. Add 1 drop of tea tree oil and mix well. Roll the tampon into this mixture, making it wet and well coated. Insert the tampon into the vagina, and leave it in place for two to three hours. Repeat as necessary. Don't use any other essential oil on a tampon but tea tree oil—it is a powerful antifungal agent and the only oil mild enough for the very delicate vaginal area. It must only be used in low dilutions.

Although I have included this tampon method in a chapter that offers help for discomforts during pregnancy, it is advisable that you do *not* insert tampons into your vagina during pregnancy. Use the external methods for easing yeast infections. However, if you have a severe yeast infection that cannot be controlled by vaginal suppositories and you wish to use this soothing method, seek the advice of your midwife or doctor *before using it.*

Tampons should also not be used during the weeks following childbirth, because of infection. Again, ask your midwife or doctor for advice.

Women who use tampons should be aware of a rare condition known as toxic shock syndrome. It is caused by a bacterium and has been found to be more common in tampon users. It can quite rapidly lead to a feverish illness; the symptoms include fever, rash, vomiting, sore throat, dizziness, and diarrhea.

Your doctor or midwife should be able to give you advice about toxic shock syndrome and the use of tampons. Generally, a tampon should never be left in place for more than three hours, and it is best not to use them at night. Also, always use the lowest-absorbency tampon you can and check that the previous tampon has been removed before inserting another.

Yeast Essential Oil Mix
In a small dropper bottle (available at the pharmacy) add about 1½ teaspoons (8 milliliters) of tea tree oil and about ⅓ teaspoon (2 milliliters) of lavender oil. Mix well.

Soothing Yeast Infection Cream
To 1 ounce (30 grams) of unperfumed cream, unperfumed gel (ask your pharmacist if unsure), or aloe gel, add 7 drops of the yeast essential oil mix.

9

Aromahelp for Labor and Birth

These days, natural childbirth has taken on a new meaning. It is no longer a taboo subject, pitting mothers against doctors and the establishment. Not so long ago mothers who did not want to be numbed with Demarol or wired to machinery during childbirth had to search for hospitals or obstetricians who did not consider their way the only way.

Today a mother is rightfully given the choice of how she wants to give birth. Views on orthodox and alternative pain relief have changed, and they can work hand in hand. Hospital staff respect the mother's preference and aim to make the birth a safe but happy experience for both mother and child. The same staff who can help perform an emergency cesarean can also be found scenting the room with jasmine or lavender and massaging the mother's back with aromatic oils.

However well you plan your labor, birth is often a very unpredictable and dramatic event. Even the strongest willed may find that their deliveries did not go as they had planned. For example, you may have planned a natural birth only to find yourself having an epidural or even a cesarean. Don't feel upset if this happens to you, and don't feel that you have failed in some way. The most important thing is that your baby is healthy and was delivered safely.

ESSENTIAL OILS FOR LABOR

If you have decided that you want the full benefits of modern medicine when you give birth, essential oils can still be of enormous help; if you want a natural childbirth, they can prove invaluable. Feedback from my clients and midwives confirms that women who get the best results from aromatherapy during labor are those who have used the oils during pregnancy. As one midwife put it, "The mothers who have used the oils before know what to expect from them and are calmed by their smell as soon as they reach the unit. They don't need to waste time grasping the concept of them, whereas mothers experiencing oils for the first time still get relief from pain with the massages but don't understand immediately that the smell of these oils can be calming at a time when they may already be in some distress." If you are planning to use essential oils at any stage of your labor—even if it is just for a soothing bath when you are still at home and in the first stage—then it is best to be familiar with them.

ROSE

Rose, the most feminine of all oils, is said to have an affinity with the reproductive system. In everyday use, it is chosen for many uterine disorders because it has a regulating, toning, and cleansing effect on the uterus. For this reason, rose is highly appropriate for labor. It is a tonic to the entire system and can assist the circulation, which in turn can encourage deep and calm breathing. Rose is renowned for its antidepressant qualities. It has a lovely, uplifting aroma that helps calm nervous feelings.

Rose can be used alone in a massage oil, but I suggest an equal blend with lavender. Or, if you are feeling totally extravagant, use it as a bath oil during the first stage of labor.

CLARY SAGE

Some people like to use clary sage during delivery because it is a great tension reliever, but some people can feel sleepy after using it. It can also be euphoric and a little too heady, and it may make everyone in the delivery room a little lightheaded. It can, however, relieve pain, so use clary sage as a compress rather than in a massage. Clary sage is not an oil I recommend if the mother has to have a general anesthetic.

NEROLI

Neroli is helpful during labor if used to reduce fear, apprehension, and anxiety. It helps you to breathe properly, allowing you to concentrate on the slow, calm breathing techniques you have practiced for labor. Just 1 or 2 drops on a tissue to inhale, or in a room spray or vaporizer, can encourage regular, rhythmic breathing.

JASMINE

Jasmine is a warm and fragrant oil that has proved to be extremely helpful during childbirth. Its analgesic and antispasmodic actions can help dull uterine pain; it strengthens contractions, which in turn helps shorten labor. Jasmine has a calming yet energizing and uplifting effect on the emotions and is an ideal oil to choose if you are feeling anxious or if your confidence needs a boost. It can also assist breathing.

I recommend using jasmine in a massage oil either by itself or in a blend with lavender, as the two oils work very well together. On its own, jasmine can also be used on a compress laid on the lower abdomen immediately after the birth to help expel the placenta.

LAVENDER

This remarkably useful oil is the one you are most likely to be offered in the hospital for pain relief. Like jasmine, lavender is very helpful in labor for dulling and easing uterine pain or for soothing aching legs and back. It increases the strength, but not the pain, of contractions. Used in a warm bath in the first stage of labor, lavender has a relaxing and calming effect, especially on the mood swings so common at this time. It will soothe headaches brought on by nervous tension and help dispel feelings of panic—so common in a first pregnancy—that result from fear of the unknown. Because of its antiseptic properties, lavender can be used in a burner, diffuser, or bowl of hot water to cleanse the air in the delivery room. Its antiseptic qualities will bring protection from germs loitering in hospital baths.

GERANIUM

Geranium is good for the circulation, which in turn will aid breathing in labor. It has a balancing effect on the emotions and a lovely uplifting smell. It is a good choice to use to scent the room during labor.

YLANG-YLANG

Ylang-ylang is a calming oil, which is why it is recommended for labor. It is soothing and acts as an antidepressant, and is particularly helpful for those with a rapid heartbeat or for those who are fearful and anxious. Ylang-ylang can help lower blood pressure and, like geranium, is a good oil to use in a burner or diffuser in the labor room.

NOTE: Many women, whether at home or in the hospital, prefer to give birth in water. I don't recommend the use of essential oils in birthing pools because the oils float in the water and there is a chance that they could get into the baby's eyes. Women who wish to give birth in water should use the oils only to scent the room.

PREPARING OILS FOR LABOR

Prepare all your labor massage and bath oils in advance. Make sure each bottle is labeled with your name and what the oil is to be used for. Keep them somewhere cool, in a plastic sponge bag to avoid leaks, and, if you need to, keep a note in your hospital suitcase to tell you where they are.

Hospitals always seem to have their heating systems on, whatever time of year, so any clothes, underwear, and nightwear you take to the hospital should be made of cotton. To refresh yourself, pack a bottle of orange flower water with some cotton balls.

LABOR DAY: THE FIRST STAGE

At last the weeks of waiting and preparation are over. During the final weeks of your pregnancy, you may well feel that your body has taken enough and you are completely fed up with the pregnant state. And, although you may be longing to see and hold your baby, you will probably feel both excited and apprehensive, or even fearful. These are perfectly natural reactions and are not just confined to women who are having a first baby. Birth is an overwhelming, all-absorbing experience every time.

Your contractions have started and you have had a "bloody show" or maybe your waters have broken. Whatever has occurred, your labor has started and you are on your way. Whether you are having your baby at home or in the hospital, you will almost certainly—unless there are medical reasons—be encouraged to keep active until the contractions are quite strong. Keeping moderately active is a good idea because it helps speed up the birth and relieve pain.

AROMAHELP

❧ If you go into labor during the early evening, use the labor bath mix (below) to soothe and relieve the tension caused by excitement and apprehension. The mix will allow you to get a few hours of sleep—very important because you have a lot of work left to do.

❧ Get your partner to massage you (see "Labor Massage" on page 79).

❧ As the contractions become stronger—whether you are still at home or in the hospital—a warm bath is a great pain reliever. If your waters have broken, check with your midwife or doctor to make sure it is all right; opinions vary, but many hospitals allow mothers to stay in the bath as long as they feel comfortable.

Labor Bath Mix
To a warm bath, add 2–3 drops of lavender oil. Swish the water to disperse the oil. Relax and soak for ten minutes.

THE ADVANCED FIRST STAGE

As the first stage progresses, whether you are at home or in the hospital, you will probably be in the very welcome and reassuring care of your midwife or doctor. During this sometimes long stage of labor, the uterine muscles are working hard at pulling up and opening the cervix. Women experience labor pains differently—some may feel pain in the lower back; others may feel pain across the lower abdomen or down the thighs.

As the contractions become stronger, you can put into practice all the relaxing techniques you have learned over the past few months. Use the help of your massage partner or willing midwife.

AROMAHELP

❧ You may find that spending long periods soaking in a bath is a great pain reliever at this stage, unless of course, there are medical reasons why you can't have a bath. Use the labor bath mix given on page 78.

🌿 A compress on the lower back or abdomen (below) will also help ease pain.

🌿 Don't just do one thing, though. Try both aromatic baths and compresses, coupled with massage and frequent changes of position. Keep moving around as much as you can during this stage of labor. It also helps to perfume the delivery room (see page 82).

Compress for Lower Back or Abdomen

To 8 ounces (240 milliliters) of warm water, add 2–3 drops of clary sage, jasmine, or lavender oil. Agitate well. Swish a clean cloth in the water, squeeze it out, and place it on either the lower back or the abdomen. Leave for as long as you feel comfortable or until the compress loses warmth. Repeat if necessary.

LABOR MASSAGE

Whenever we experience pain, our natural instinct is to rub it better. Nowhere could this apply more than in labor. Deep, firm, rhythmic massage can greatly reduce and relieve labor pains, especially in the first stage of labor when you may still be at home. By the time you go into labor, your partner should be familiar with how you like to be massaged. Get him to practice the movements below well before arriving at the delivery room. Massage during labor is without a doubt a great relief; it is even better with essential oils.

If you have no one to accompany you to the hospital to give you an aromatherapy massage and you would like to use essential oils for your birth, find out well in advance the policy in the delivery unit. Inquire about midwives who use essential oils. If no one who is sympathetic to or familiar with them is certain to be on duty when you give birth, determine whether others will understand your needs and be willing to massage you and prepare a room oil or compress if you want one. You will probably find someone who is more than happy to help you, but it is worth checking in advance. If your partner is attending the birth, it would also be courteous to let the midwives know if you intend to use essential oils in your birth plan.

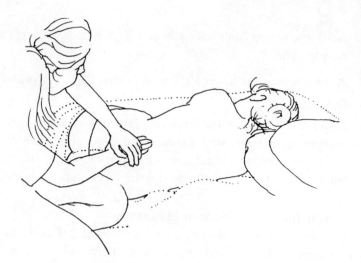

How to Give a Massage During Labor

If you will be massaging a mother-to-be, comforting movements for labor include the following (use the labor day massage oil on page 81):

🌸 Use deep, firm, circular pressure around the lower back. Press the heel of your hand into the lower back of the mother-to-be.

🌸 Use pressure with the thumbs in the center of each buttock. Press and release several times. Firm pressure with the heel of your hand in her sacral area (the area below the spine) brings comfort. Massage firmly in circular movements. This is a method she will probably want to return to throughout her labor.

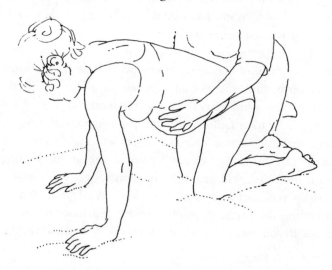

The mother-to-be may feel like sitting astride a chair (as she did in pregnancy massage) so the back and shoulders can be massaged easily, or she may want to change her position frequently. If she is comfortable on all fours, gently rocking from side to side may give relief. Kneel behind her and massage in gentle circular movements down the sides of the abdomen from where the top of the stomach begins to the thighs and up again. Repeat this for as long as she wants.

Massaging her feet, by pressing quite firmly into the soles with circular movements, is very comforting. Use one hand to grip the top of the foot over the instep to steady it; use the other hand on the same foot, pressing firmly into the middle of the sole. Make circular movements, varying the pressure; squeeze and release the foot. These movements should all be repeated several times.

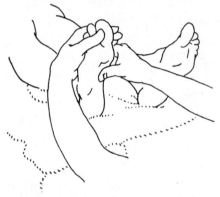

Still with one hand steadying the foot, press with the thumb of the other hand up and down the foot in an imaginary line. Press and release, varying the pressure and time spent on each foot according to her wishes. This feels good if the press–release action is done in circular movements.

Still on the feet, with both hands well oiled, massage all over the top and sole of the foot and lower leg, letting the fingers circle around the ankles.

Labor Day Massage Oil

To 2½ tablespoons (50 milliliters) of almond oil, add 6 drops of lavender oil and 6 drops of jasmine oil. Jasmine is quite indulgent to use because it is so expensive. If you can't afford jasmine, just use lavender on its own.

PERFUMING THE DELIVERY ROOM

Essential oils in the delivery room will help keep the mother and everyone around her sane. For the baby, to come into the world into a sweetly scented room that is relaxed, welcoming, and happy must be the perfect way to be born.

Essential oils help kill airborne bacteria and any stale unpleasant odors in the room; they also help the mother feel calm, relaxed, and happy. But take care: Essential oils are very strong and you don't want the midwife floating around the room in a trance.

Oils for the Delivery Room

To a bowl of hot water, add 3 drops of your favorite oil or a mix of two of the following: lavender (relaxing and antiseptic), bergamot (a great antidepressant), geranium (very uplifting), or lemon (very refreshing and good if the mother is tired after a long labor).

THE TRANSITION STAGE

The transition stage is really the end of the first stage of labor, when the cervix has not yet fully opened and you have been told not to start pushing, although you may want to. During the transition stage, some women find they begin to shake, especially in their legs. It can be helpful if your (by now long-suffering) partner can massage your legs quite firmly, as this seems to steady them. But be forewarned—this is a very unpredictable and dramatic stage of labor and you may find you don't want anything to do with anyone. Don't worry if you shout and lose your temper with anything that moves—including your partner. It is quite normal and birth attendants are used to it. In fact, it's a sure sign that the second stage is imminent.

AROMAHELP

Some women find a cloth soaked in cool water wiped over the face and neck refreshing and calming. Add 2 drops of either rose, neroli, or lavender oil to a bowl of cool water. Soak a washcloth in the water and use it to mop the face.

THE SECOND STAGE

In the second stage of labor, the cervix is fully dilated. The feel of the pains changes as the intense urge to push takes over. Calm, controlled breathing will help you over the top "wave" of the contractions and will mean that you have plenty of puff left to push with. If you find your breathing becoming erratic, sniff one or two drops of neroli on a tissue to calm you and prevent overbreathing. Between contractions, try to relax. As you feel the next contraction coming, it helps to imagine the beginning of the pain as being like a large approaching wave. Imagine that your body is in total control of this wave. As the pain increases, visualize the wave gradually rising to full height, reaching its peak, and being held there briefly; then letting go, slowly falling to a flat level, and tapering off at the water's edge, as the pain decreases and fades away.

AROMAHELP

- Massage can still be soothing, but you will probably be too busy for one at this stage of labor.

- A calming cloth for your partner to dab your face with will probably be very welcome. To a bowl of warm water, add 2–3 drops of lavender oil. Dip a washcloth or other suitable cloth into the water and use it to mop up any perspiration or to give a soothing dab to the face.

- Place 1–2 drops of mandarin, petitgrain, neroli, ylang-ylang, or geranium oil on a tissue and inhale when needed. This may make your breathing easier and will certainly make you feel more cheerful. If you find your breathing becoming erratic during this stage, neroli oil is particularly recommended because it is very calming and will prevent hyperventilation when gaspy breaths release carbon dioxide too quickly, making you feel dizzy and panicky with a tingling face and limbs.

- Add 2–3 drops of neroli, ylang-ylang, or geranium oil to a bowl of hot water in the delivery room. This will give a calming scent to the room. Make sure the bowl is placed somewhere out of the way of the proceedings.

THE BIRTH AND THIRD STAGE

All the past hours of work and effort seem forgotten as a somewhat slippery baby is placed on your abdomen. You will probably feel so overwhelmed that the third stage of labor—the delivery of the placenta—will probably go unnoticed by you. Relax and enjoy these moments of getting to know each other. You will always remember them.

AROMAHELP

❧ When the baby has been delivered, a compress can help expel the placenta. This is more likely to happen at a home delivery. To a bowl of warm water, add 2–3 drops of jasmine oil. Agitate the water well, wring out a washcloth or other suitable cloth, and place the compress over the lower abdomen. As the compress loses heat, replace it with another. Leave it in position until the placenta is delivered.

❧ After the two of you have been washed and tidied up, you will probably be expected to sleep for a while. I was always far too excited to sleep after giving birth. If this happens to you, sprinkle a few drops of neroli or lavender oil onto a tissue and inhale the aroma. Then just lie back on the pillow, close your eyes, and relax. You might even be able to get some sleep.

Postpartum Care and Adjusting to Motherhood

Along with the relief that the labor is over and, hopefully, all is well, there may be some minor discomforts after the birth. After all, your body has taken a substantial battering. Aromatherapy can help you in conjunction with whatever help you receive in the hospital or from your midwife. In fact, natural products are regaining popularity in maternity units. But if you are in doubt about using anything, first check with your midwife. Remember to take your postpartum aromatherapy kit with you to the hospital.

HEALING THE PERINEUM

If the perineum (the skin between the vagina and the anus) has stitches after an episiotomy or tearing during the birth, you are bound to feel somewhat sore. Essential oils can help.

As soon as your midwife agrees, add essential oils to the bath or bidet. The mixture below will help prevent infection, heal wounds, and encourage new skin to grow. Use the formula even if you don't have stitches—it will help to prevent infection in the days following the birth.

To a warm bath, add 2 drops of lavender oil and 2 drops of cypress oil. Swish the water to mix the oil in. Relax and soak for ten to fifteen minutes. Follow this procedure up to three times a day while soreness persists.

CESAREAN DELIVERY

Expect to feel tired after a cesarean. Not only do you have a baby to look after, but you are also recovering from an operation. Allow yourself extra time to get back to normal.

Don't compare yourself to other cesarean mothers. For every one who leaps out of bed and walks with a straight back three days after delivery, there will be ten more who will only be able to shuffle along, bent over and clutching the wound across their lower abdomens. Everyone has their own rate of recovery, so don't worry. Most mothers are able to walk upright by the end of a week, but you should give yourself at least six months to get fit again.

Don't spend time worrying that your birth didn't go as you planned or feeling that you failed because you had a cesarean. No one is judging you apart from yourself.

AROMAHELP

As soon as you are allowed to take a bath, add 4 drops of lavender oil to warm (never hot) water. Swish to disperse the oil. Relax and soak for ten to fifteen minutes. Lavender will help you relax and help your wound heal more quickly.

POSTPARTUM BLUES

It is quite normal to feel tired and weepy for a couple of days after the birth. This is often called "third-day tears" or "milk blues" because it coincides with the arrival of breast milk. Once again, the hormones are to blame for this, so don't be alarmed if the smallest things makes you burst into tears.

It is also a bit of a shock for first-time mothers to cope with leaking breasts, a sore bottom, and—if all that weren't enough—a baby as well! It would be enough to make anyone cry. These postpartum blues usually clear up after a few days; it's some assurance that they are never quite as bad with the second baby, if only because you know what to expect. It is also worth bearing in mind that the days leading up to and following the birth were probably quite exciting, even if some of the proceedings were unpleasant. You probably received a tremendous amount of attention from medical staff, friends, and family, then, suddenly, you are home on your own and looking after your baby. No one prepares you or tells you what it's like to suddenly be so totally responsible for a tiny human being, one who has been part of you for the last nine months but whom you now have to get to know all over again. In addition to the excitement and love this new responsibility brings, it can also bring some frightening feelings. A week or so after the birth of my first child I remember thinking I would never be able to do anything on the spur of the moment again. I was actually quite scared. I didn't realize that, although the responsibilities that come with being a mother would always be there, a child isn't always going to be a helpless babe-in-arms.

AROMAHELP

🌿 An aromatic bath will help chase away any depressing feelings, so use any offers of help to look after the baby and take yourself off to the bathroom. Enjoy the freedom of being able to lie in the bath without looking like a hippo anymore and without a pair of feet pressing on your ribs from the inside. If you have time, wash your hair as well. Many mothers say they feel better afterward. To the bathwater (warm, never hot), add up to 5 drops of any of the following: ylang-ylang, bergamot, jasmine, neroli, or clary sage oil. These are all oils that can help lift your mood and make you feel more relaxed and cheerful. Swish the water to disperse the oil. Relax and soak for ten to fifteen minutes.

🌿 Some hospitals and midwives advise showers rather than baths for a few days after the birth. If you have been advised to shower, wash as usual, then add 2–3 drops of either ylang-ylang, bergamot, jasmine, neroli, or clary sage oil to a wet sponge and rub over your body while breathing in the vapors.

🎶 If you can't bathe or shower, sprinkle 1–2 drops of either ylang-ylang, bergamot, jasmine, neroli, or clary sage oil onto a tissue and sniff the uplifting aromas. Take care to keep the tissue away from the baby.

🎶 If you are really suffering after the birth, there is a very special pick-me-up using oil from different parts of the orange tree— neroli from the flowers, petitgrain from the leaves and twigs, and orange from the fruit (below). It is particularly helpful for those suffering from postpartum depression because the very wholeness of the tree helps make them feel complete.

Special Pick-Me-Up

To a warm bath, add 2 drops of neroli, 2 drops of petitgrain, and 2 drops of orange oil. Or make a very special massage oil by adding 2 drops of neroli, 2 drops of petitgrain, and 2 drops of orange oil to 2½ tablespoons (50 milliliters) of sweet almond oil.

POSTPARTUM FATIGUE AND ADJUSTING TO MOTHERHOOD

Sometimes a mother can continue to feel emotionally and physically drained for quite a while after the birth. She may be unable to concentrate on day-to-day tasks, and with the baby taking all her time, life seems all baby. The days take on a pattern of complete nonachievement.

We can joke about the prospect of broken nights before the birth, but no one really knows what it's like until they experience it. To be waked at two or four in the morning, especially when someone next to you is happily snoring, is not fun. A small tip: I recommend keeping a baby that is on regular night feeding in his or her crib beside your bed. The baby can then be picked up and fed without you having to move from bed, and it's comforting for both of you to be near each other.

If this is your first baby, you may wonder how you will ever have the time or energy to resume life as it was before, but take heart. Your body has just completed several months of the most important job it will ever do, so give yourself a pat on the back.

Follow these tips:

- Take time to recover at your own pace—not someone else's. If you are planning to go back to work, make sure you feel fit enough and are happy with the child-care arrangements. I see many women in my treatment rooms who have gone back to work too early and are feeling run down and tired.

- Forget the housework. If the cobwebs have cobwebs, it doesn't matter, and if anyone else in the house is bothered about it, direct them to the cleaning materials. Gratefully accept all offers of help with the chores.

- Look after yourself, eat a well-balanced diet, and allow yourself time to rest with your feet up during the day while the baby sleeps. If you have other children, keep them occupied in the same room that you are in, even if it is just watching television, so that you can keep an eye on them and don't have to keep rushing out to see what they are up to.

- Make sure you get exercise and fresh air, even if it means just taking the baby out for a walk every day. Research has shown that exercise can release hormones that ward off melancholy feelings and depression. The fresh air is good for the baby too.

- As soon as you can, get out with your partner again, even if it's just for an hour.

- Give yourself a treat: get your hair done, buy something new to wear, ask a friend to lunch (preferably one who will arrive at your house with the entire contents of a deli counter).

AROMAHELP

- An aromatherapy massage using oils with tonic properties will help you get back to normal. Not only will it help you relax and feel good, but it will keep the skin on the stomach, legs, and breasts well moisturized, which will encourage suppleness and tone while your weight returns to normal. It will also encourage restful sleep, even between night feedings. One desperate and tired mother reported the best night's sleep she'd had in five years after receiving a massage. In many Eastern countries, women routinely receive massage after childbirth to help the abdomen get back to normal.

Obviously, it is better to receive an aromatherapy massage from a professional, but the next best thing is a massage from a willing partner or friend. Follow the basic plan for pregnancy massage (see page 51), but ask your partner to avoid the abdominal area altogether if there is any tenderness or if there is still postpartum bleeding. Don't massage anywhere near a cesarean scar. A back massage is particularly relaxing because the back is under a lot of stress and strain during pregnancy; the shoulders can ache after breast- or bottle-feeding, especially with a heavy baby (make sure you are well supported with cushions when you breast-feed). Use the postpartum massage oil described below.

❧ If you are having trouble sleeping, slip into a warm bath before bed. Add 3 drops of either lavender, marjoram, or Roman chamomile oil to the water. Alternatively, try any of the oils recommended for postpartum blues: ylang-ylang, bergamot, jasmine, neroli, or clary sage. Swish the water to disperse the oil. Relax and soak for ten to fifteen minutes.

❧ For a refreshing morning bath that will set you up for the day, add 2–3 drops of either geranium or bergamot oil and 2–3 drops of rosemary oil to the warm water. Swish the water to disperse the oil and soak as usual for ten to fifteen minutes.

❧ You can use oils around the house to scent the rooms. To a bowl of hot water, a fragrancer, or a burner, add 2–4 drops of any of the recommended postpartum oils: petitgrain, geranium, mandarin, rose, bergamot, ylang-ylang, lemon, lavender, or rosemary. All of them are refreshing, but a particularly cheering and lovely blend you may want to try is geranium and lemon.

Postpartum Massage Oil
To 1¼ tablespoons (25 milliliters) of carrier oil, add 3 drops of lavender oil, 3 drops of rosemary oil, and 3 drops of geranium oil. Or try a mix of any of the following oils: petitgrain, geranium, mandarin, rose, bergamot, ylang-ylang, lavender, or rosemary. If you are breast-feeding, use only 1–2 drops of essential oil to every teaspoon (5 milliliters) of carrier oil. Essential oils are very strong and can be passed through in breast milk.

POSTPARTUM DEPRESSION

Many women suffer from postpartum blues or fatigue, symptoms that with time and rest usually fade after a few weeks. But in true postpartum depression, the feelings of fatigue, exhaustion from lack of sleep, and anxiety are joined by other physical and emotional problems that can range from fears about being a "bad" mother to resentment toward a partner, sexual anxieties, or feeling you're a failure if you can't breastfeed. Sometimes these problems don't appear until many months after the birth and can have their roots in a variety of causes.

These feelings are often birth-related. Some women are disappointed and unhappy about their deliveries and are left feeling dissatisfied. They may think their performance at the birth wasn't up to the expectations they'd set for themselves. One woman described this feeling as one of utter desolation; another said she couldn't get over the disappointment of having to have a cesarean. Someone else felt that after what she described as two physically and mentally unsatisfying births, she had to have another child to experience birth satisfaction. She did this with her third baby and then said that she felt complete.

If you have any such worries about yourself or your baby, talk to your midwife or doctor. They are there to help you, and they are able to spot severe postpartum depression before it becomes a long-term or severe problem. It also helps to talk about your fears with other mothers, many of whom experience the same feelings to a greater or lesser degree.

Aromatherapy has a part to play in postpartum depression. If you can, see an aromatherapist as well as your doctor.

11

Breast-Feeding

It must be the most natural thing in the world for a mother to put her newborn baby to her breast. There are many advantages to breast-feeding: breast milk is a perfect, balanced food for a baby; breast milk is free and readily available; and breast-feeding increases the bond with your baby.

During the first few days after birth, the breasts produce a watery fluid, colostrum, which contains antibodies that can protect the baby from infection. Even if you decide to give up breast-feeding after a few weeks, you will still have given your baby a good start by passing these antibodies through breast milk.

INCREASING THE MILK SUPPLY

Sometimes your breasts will not provide the constant supply of milk you were hoping for, and often, especially with new mothers, breast-feeding isn't as easy as expected. In fact, both you and your baby have to "learn" how to breast-feed, a process that can take quite a few days. The following tips may help:

❧ Try to keep a relaxed attitude about feeding. It won't benefit you or the baby if you get tense, and you can hinder the "let-down reflex"—the tingly feeling in and around the nipple that indicates that the milk is ready to flow. This sensation has been described as feeling rather like the nose does just before a sneeze. It can feel unpleasant at first, but it settles down to a light tingle after the first few weeks.

- The more you put the baby to your breast, the more milk you will produce. It's what's known as supply and demand. During the early days, it will seem as if your breasts have taken on a new status in life!

- Don't be discouraged. Just let the baby feed whenever he or she needs to, and you will soon establish a good supply. Breast-fed babies will need to be fed more often than bottle-fed babies.

- Don't feel that your initial experience is how breast-feeding will be all the time. It won't. You may not believe this when you are trying to cope with heavy, leaking breasts and elephant-size bras, but after the first few weeks everything will settle down—the size of your breasts will decrease, you will lose some lumpiness, your breasts will stop leaking, and you will be able to put your baby to the breast anytime without fuss or bother.

- Don't get too tired because it will affect the amount of milk you produce. Try to rest as much as you can, and snatch sleep when the baby sleeps, even if it happens to be midafternoon.

- As a bonus, this is the one time in your life when you can eat pretty much what you want. You will use up plenty of calories supplying the baby with milk and still lose the weight gained during pregnancy.

- You will need to take in plenty of fluid. I found that a large glass of springwater half an hour before each feeding, plus another glass afterward, worked well. Drinking fennel tea can increase the milk flow.

- Wear a comfortable bra day and night to support the breasts. Until the milk supply settles down, you may need to wear disposable breast pads to help with the leaking.

- If you continue to have problems, contact La Leche League for the telephone number of the nearest counselor. They can supply help and advice and lend breast pumps (see appendix 1 for addresses).

AROMAHELP

Use the standard pregnancy massage oil (see page 53) on the breasts daily to help keep the breasts supple and prevent stretch marks. Even if you didn't get stretch marks during pregnancy, the breasts may still be susceptible to them because of their increased or fluctuating size. Continue to use the oil twice daily until your breasts return to normal size or until you discontinue breast-feeding altogether. Remember, though, to wash any oil off the nipple before feeding or clean with a moistened cotton ball and then pat dry. Medical opinion is that the breasts should not be washed too frequently when breast-feeding, but it's best not to have any gel or cream on the breast before you feed. This also applies to any creams you may have been given by your doctor.

ENGORGED BREASTS

Every woman who has breast-fed remembers the feeling of waking up with rock-hard, aching breasts. The best cure is to feed the baby, but because engorgement usually occurs during the first week of breast-feeding, it may mean that a very new, sleepy baby won't be able to empty each breast completely. In the beginning, the breasts can become full and lumpy very quickly, perhaps well before the baby needs another feeding. Your midwife or doctor may suggest expressing the milk with a pump.

AROMAHELP

🍂 Try taking a hot bath with 2 drops of lavender oil and 2 drops of geranium oil added to the water. Swish to disperse the oils, then lie back and let the water cover your breasts. Or soak a washcloth in the water and hold it to your breasts. You will find that this procedure relieves the pressure and decongests the breasts.

🍂 Also try using a compress. A hot compress will relieve pressure; a cold compress will reduce swelling. Use whichever is most suitable. To 8 ounces (240 milliliters) of either hot or cold water, add 2 drops of lavender oil and 2 drops of geranium oil. Soak a clean cloth in the water, squeeze it, and hold it to the breasts. You can then try to gently express some milk.

SORE NIPPLES

Sometimes the baby may not take the area surrounding the nipple (the areola) into his or her mouth when feeding but instead just suck at the nipple. Not only will this make the baby frustrated at not getting enough milk, but it will make your nipples very sore. You may also get cracked nipples.

Ask your midwife or doctor to help you position the baby properly. Don't worry about having to ask for help—nearly every mother needs help with breast-feeding at first. Nipple shields through which the baby can suck are available at any pharmacy and may help until the soreness has abated.

AROMAHELP

If you have soreness around the nipples, make up the sore nipple gel (below) and apply it to the nipples and areola after feeding the baby. Remember to wipe or wash the nipples to remove any remaining gel before feeding again—babies must not get essential oils in their mouths.

Sore Nipple Gel

To 1 tablespoon (20 milliliters) of aloe gel, add 3 drops of rose oil and 1 drop of benzoin oil. Or to 1 tablespoon (20 milliliters) of aloe gel, add ½ tablespoon (10 milliliters) of a calendula carrier oil.

MASTITIS

Milk can block the ducts and lead to lumpy breasts and mastitis, a condition in which the breasts become hot and inflamed. Don't stop breast-feeding if this happens—the breasts need to be emptied—but speak to your doctor or midwife, particularly if you are feeling unwell, because the breasts may have become infected.

AROMAHELP

Bathe the breasts in warm water to which you have added 2 drops of lavender oil and 2 drops of geranium oil, or use the compress method described for sore breasts (see page 68). Repeat every few hours until the condition clears.

12

✤

Getting Back Into Shape

There are a few lucky women who sail through their pregnancies and labors and effortlessly resume life again with figures and complexions that are seemingly untouched by any of the hormonal upheaval of the past nine months. The other 99 percent of us, however, need a little help boosting our postpregnancy morale.

Because the body works as a whole, everything we do to one part of it will have an effect on the entire body. After the baby is born, diet, exercise, rest, calmness of mind, and a simple beauty routine will all work together, however gradually, to help you feel totally restored and to help you regain your confidence. But don't push yourself too hard. Let your body take its own time to get back into shape.

AROMAHELP

🌿 For three months after the birth, try to schedule regular treatments with an aromatherapist, or ask a friend or your partner to give you a regular massage, even just a foot massage (see pages 26, 54, and 81).

🌿 Continue with essential bath oils and experiment with them (remember to use only 4 drops in the bath if you are breast-feeding).

🎵 Continue to use anti-stretch-mark oil (see page 69) on your body while it is returning to normal because you can still get stretch marks while your body is decreasing in weight.

GETTING YOUR FIGURE BACK INTO SHAPE

Do not expect your body to spring back to its prepregnancy state immediately after the birth. It usually takes about three or four weeks for the uterus to return to its normal size. Your doctor or midwife will check your uterus at your six-week postpartum checkup. The stretched muscles and skin of your abdominal area will need both time and exercise to recover completely. Expect to carry excess weight around your hips, thighs, and upper arms for a while. You may also suffer from fluid retention—which will soon dissipate—and cellulite as a result of the hormonal changes. Just remember that it took you nine months to get to the size you were for the birth of your baby; don't expect to get back into shape again in nine days. With time and few simple measures, you will.

DIET

Don't vow to starve yourself back into your jeans within six weeks. You will probably feel tired in the weeks following the birth, and you need to regain your strength now more than ever. A low-calorie intake is the last thing your body needs, especially if you are breast-feeding, because you need calories to produce a good supply of milk. One of the bonuses of breast-feeding, though, is that it helps the body get back into shape naturally. If you diet, you will not feel well; if you don't feel well, you will not look well, and you could become trapped in a vicious circle.

Everyone recovers their energy at different rates, but give yourself at least three months. Just be careful about what you eat in what I call the "after-delivery period." Think of your diet as a way of life rather than as weight loss. Whether you are breast-feeding or not, try to eat a well-balanced diet. You can lose weight without starving or depriving yourself of the occasional chocolate bar. Making a few of the following simple changes to your eating habits will help:

🎵 Aim for a good, balanced diet with lots of vitamin-rich fruit and leafy green vegetables; plenty of low-fat protein foods such as chicken, fish, or legumes; yogurt; and carbohydrates such as cereals, whole-grain breads, and potatoes. Remember that carbohydrate foods are not fattening in themselves; it is just the sugar, jam, or butter often eaten with them that pushes up the calorie content.

❧ Try to cut back on your overall fat intake (by trimming fat from meat and avoiding oily or fried foods) and cut back on sugary foods.

❧ Salt can contribute to fluid retention, so cut back on your salt intake. Try herbs instead or use a salt substitute for flavoring.

❧ Ready-prepared or processed foods will seem like a godsend, but try to limit them. Check the contents list on the packages for salt, sugar, and hidden fats as well as for unwanted additives.

❧ Drink plenty of water. Apart from the extra fluid breast-feeding mothers need, we all need at least eight glasses a day to flush out the system and keep the skin clear and well hydrated.

❧ If you are hungry (and you will be quite a lot of the time if you are breast-feeding), snack on fruit or yogurts between meals rather than cookies, candy, or cake. If you normally consume chocolate or cookies aim to be realistic and initially limit them rather than cut them out altogether.

EXERCISE

❧ To help you fully recover from the birth, a certain amount of exercise is essential, not just to burn up calories and tone you up but to improve your general well-being and to help you feel less tired. Exercise increases the blood circulation, which in turn will help the condition of the skin.

❧ Choose exercises that can fit with your daily routine. If you went to a gym or exercise class before the birth, then take it up again (once your doctor or midwife agrees you are ready and you feel strong enough). Or your exercise could be as simple as regular walking or pushing the baby carriage. If you have no one to look after the baby while you attend a regular exercise class, then try to find a class in your area that welcomes babies or take turns babysitting another mother's child so you both get the chance for an hour off every so often. Many health clubs and swimming pools offer special postpartum sessions for new mothers.

In the early days after the birth, don't neglect pelvic-floor and abdominal exercises. Strong abdominal muscles help prevent low backache, and pelvic-floor exercises are vitally important to help stretched muscles around the vagina, bladder, and anus tone up again. Neglect them and you could develop stress incontinence— a bladder that can leak when you sneeze or run for the bus. Tightening up these muscles will also mean that making love is more enjoyable—a good enough reason on its own. So however busy you are, aim to take some time every day for doing sit-ups, pelvic-floor exercises, or any other form of exercise that will tone the stomach and pelvic floor. Even as little as ten minutes a day, done regularly, will make a difference.

BODY CREAMS AND LOTIONS

In my aromatherapy treatment rooms I make up a variety of moisturizing and nourishing body and hand creams for my clients. Unlike most beauty products on the market, these creams work on individual skin problems, right down to the lower layer of the skin. You can benefit from individually tailored products at home by using unperfumed creams and adding the essential oils for your skin type.

PREPARING BODY CREAMS

When buying unperfumed creams or lotions, make sure they don't contain lanolin, which can aggravate skin rashes. Ask your local pharmacist to recommend a cream if you're unsure (or to find one by mail order, refer to appendix 1).

If the cream is in a plastic bottle, you will need to buy some glass jars (ask your pharmacist), since essential oils don't react well with plastic. Sterilize the jars by boiling before using them and make sure they are dry by putting them in a low oven. Also sterilize a small, thin-stemmed plastic utensil for mixing the creams, or boil a teaspoon for five minutes to sterilize it.

When making up body creams at home, I suggest you stick to a 1 percent dilution of the essential oils. For example a 1 percent dilution of 2 ounces (50 grams) of cream would contain 12 drops of essential oil. A 1 percent dilution of 1¼ ounces (30 grams) of cream would contain 7 drops of essential oil.

Following these directions for quantities, squeeze the cream into the jar and add the essential oils. Stir very well to make sure the oil is distributed evenly, and don't forget to label the jar afterward.

I think the fragrance is more alluring when just a single oil is used instead of a blend of several. Any of the following oils will make delicious-smelling body creams: ylang-ylang, mandarin, geranium, rose, jasmine, neroli, lavender, petitgrain, and sandalwood. See "Body Scrubs" below to determine the oils that are suitable for particular skin types. Use creams as often as you wish but preferably at least once a day.

BODY SCRUBS

The skin is one of the organs of elimination for the body, and when it is clogged up, the pores must work much harder to get rid of unwanted toxins and waste. The skin will be more receptive to oils or creams if it is not congested with dead cells, which can linger, giving skin a sallow or dull tone. By removing dead cells, the skin is thoroughly cleansed and the pores are unclogged of dirt, allowing the skin to breathe again. Skin brushing or using exfoliating scrubs gives nature a hand in this process and leaves the skin glowing and soft.

The frequency with which you use a body scrub will depend on how you think your skin looks and the time you have available, but aim for at least once a week to help a sluggish circulation. If you have had a cesarean, you must keep clear of the abdomen until the scar and any internal bruising have healed.

There are many commercially available body scrubs, but most tend to be expensive and too abrasive. The gentle scrub described below is easily made at home, with essential oils added to suit the condition of the skin (for a more detailed discussion of skin types, see page 106).

Basic Scrub Mix
Mix together 4 ounces (100 grams) of oatmeal and 4 ounces (100 grams) of ground almonds. If you only have whole almonds, first remove the skins and make sure they are dry or they will go bad when stored; then grind with a food processor. Store the mixture in a glass jar and keep the lid on to keep it dry.

USING BODY SCRUBS

Place 1–2 tablespoons of the basic scrub mix (page 100) in a small basin. Add 4 drops of a chosen essential oil, either a recommended postpartum oil or one recommended for your skin type (see below). Add ½ teaspoonful of jojoba or almond oil. Mix to a paste. Add more jojoba or almond oil if it is too stiff.

Bathe or shower as normal and pat yourself nearly dry; with damp skin, rub the paste all over your body starting at the feet and working upward (it is best to do this while standing in the bath or shower). Work the mixture into the body with gentle circular movements, avoiding areas that are sore (such as breasts or nipples), scarred areas, or areas around varicose veins. Work well into areas of cellulite or dry skin. Rinse well. The skin should be soft and glowing.

Recommended postpartum oils: Benzoin, clary sage, Roman chamomile, marjoram, rosemary, and grapefruit are best.

For dry or sensitive skin: Rose, sandalwood, and neroli are best. Other suitable oils are Roman chamomile, jasmine, and ylang-ylang.

For normal skin: Lavender, geranium, and neroli are best. Other suitable oils are sandalwood, rose, and jasmine.

For oily skin: Ylang-Ylang, geranium, lemon, lavender, and cypress are best. Another suitable oil is sandalwood.

For allergic skin: Chamomile and sandalwood are best.

GETTING RID OF CELLULITE

The body tends to use the hips and thighs as a dumping ground for surplus wastes and toxins, giving rise to the familiar orange-peel skin known as cellulite. The skin is dimply and lumpy, usually feels cold to the touch, and can be quite painful when pressed. Women tend to accumulate cellulite at times of hormonal fluctuations and are therefore far more prone to it during pregnancy.

Cellulite can affect those who are thin as often as it affects those who are overweight. It occurs when the body's elimination processes aren't functioning properly. In addition to hormonal changes (which explain the appearance of cellulite at puberty, pregnancy, and menopause), other causes of cellulite are constipation, lack of exercise, fatigue, and filling the body with toxins over a long period. These toxins include alcohol, tobacco, tea, coffee, animal fats, dairy products, and so on. Cellulite goes hand in hand with having poor circulation and poor lymphatic drainage.

An aromatherapist can help with cellulite, but I wouldn't recommend treatment until six months after the birth. To make a concentrated effort to remove cellulite involves a very strict detoxification diet and may include a lymph drainage program. Neither is advisable until you are fully healed, especially if you are breast-feeding.

In the meantime, there are specific measures you can take to reduce cellulite:

❦ Exercise and diet improvement are the first steps. Follow the instructions given in the sections on diet and exercise (see pages 97–99). The measures mentioned there, such as cutting back on fat intake and drinking plenty of water to flush toxins out of the system, will help. It is also important to get some form of regular exercise. It should be gentle, especially if you are still fragile or tired after the birth. Swimming, cycling, and walking regularly are ideal. The jerky movements of jogging or skipping, though, have not been shown to improve the condition of cellulite.

❦ Dry skin brushing will also help. It is a practice used by natural practitioners to help cleanse the body of unreleased toxins. It stimulates the circulation and lymphatic systems and encourages the body's elimination systems to release wastes, thus breaking down determined fatty deposits.

DRY SKIN BRUSHING

Brushing the skin with a stiff, dry brush—preferably of natural bristle—encourages the removal of dead skin cells, unblocks the pores, and helps the body eliminate wastes. It is an invigorating procedure, one that will make the skin glow by removing dry, scaly skin. Done regularly, there will be a gradual reduction in cellulite and the legs and thighs will improve in tone and shape.

Dry skin brushing must be done every day before a bath, preferably in the morning. In the evening dry skin brushing can be too stimulating for the body, and you may find you can't sleep afterward.

Remember to brush very, very gently to begin with. The instructions below indicate the number of times you should brush—these are the times you should work up to, not begin with. Always brush with

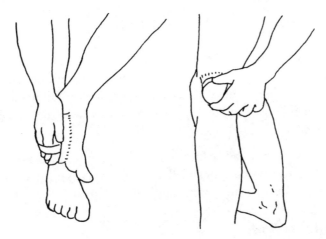

long, firm strokes. If the brush is very scratchy, soak it overnight to soften the bristles. Always remember to wash it frequently.

❧ Brush one leg at a time, starting with the sole of the foot. Brush the sole, continue over the foot, up to the knee, and all around the leg. Do this about four times.

❧ Continue up the knee and along the thigh to the buttocks, where you can brush in circular movements and a little harder.

❧ Brush the arms starting at the hands, between each finger, working from the wrist to the elbow and then up to the shoulder. To help the lymph glands under the arms, brush there in circular movements, five times one way and then five times the other. Then brush the neck and back.

❧ Avoid the breasts, but brush the chest. Go a little more slowly and gently over the trunk and abdomen, working around the lower abdomen in a clockwise direction because the large bowel works in that direction.

CAUTION: However beneficial skin brushing is, it is not a treatment I would recommend during the early days of lactation. During this time and until your baby is at least eight weeks old, it is better to cleanse the body with a gentle body scrub (see page 100). Skin brushing is a very stimulating treatment and will encourage the body to leak milk.

AROMAHELP

※ In the first few months after the birth I recommend a daily body scrub; from at least two months after the birth. I recommend daily skin brushing. These procedures should be followed by an anticellulite bath and then perhaps a massage with the anticellulite massage oil (below).

※ If you have very bad cellulite more than six months after the birth, it is worth visiting a qualified aromatherapist (see appendix 1 to find one in your area) who can help you to deal with it.

Anticellulite Bath
To a warm bath, add 2–3 drops of either rosemary, cypress, or geranium oil. Swish water to disperse oil. Soak in the water for ten to fifteen minutes.

Anticellulite Massage Oil
To 2½ tablespoons (50 milliliters) of sweet almond oil or grapeseed oil, add 4 drops of geranium oil, 4 drops of cypress oil, and 3 drops of rosemary oil. Mix well. Use at least three times a week, after a bath.

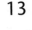

13

Postpregnancy Skin and Hair

After the hormonal ups and downs of pregnancy and birth, the condition of your skin can temporarily change. Even if it is usually problem-free, it may become dry, oily, or even prone to pimples. Essential oils can make a big difference to postpregnancy skin when they become part of a daily routine. The oils penetrate the skin, sinking deep into the lower layers and getting to work on the cells there before they start their journey to the skin's surface. It takes three weeks for new, well-conditioned cells to reach the top layer of skin (although as we age, the process takes longer). So if you have a special date, book an appointment with an aromatherapist three weeks in advance, and be vigilant about using essential oils for a daily facial massage (see page 107).

The condition of the hair can also change, sometimes dramatically, during and after pregnancy. Normally bouncy and problem-free hair can become dank and oily. Just as with the skin, aromatherapy can help restore the condition of postpregnancy hair.

POSTPREGNANCY SKIN

It would be foolish to expect any new (or not so new) mother to perform an elaborate and time-consuming daily beauty ritual. You will probably find that you have less time for yourself now than you've ever had in your life. If this is your first baby, this realization can be something of a shock. If your skin is suffering, it's important to find a simple routine that is easy to stick to. There is no need to try all the suggestions I make below. Just pick out what appeals to you. The great bonus of essential oils is that not only can they be added to carrier oils, they can be incorporated into any perfumed creams or lotions you already use. Here are a few general tips:

🎝 For the first three to four weeks after the baby is born, you will probably be too tired at night to do anything more strenuous than have a quick wash or bath (don't forget to add essential oils to the water to help you relax and sleep). However tired you feel, don't be tempted to get into bed without taking your makeup off—that is, if you've had time to put it on in the first place. Cleanse your face and splash several times with tepid water to close the pores. Tone with either rose water (available at the pharmacist) if your skin is dry to normal, or orange flower water if your skin is oily or a combination skin.

🎝 After a bath or shower, continue to use the anti-stretch-mark oil (see page 69). It will not only help keep your skin soft and supple, it will help prevent stretch marks that can form as your body shrinks back to its normal size. The citrus smell is also cheerfully uplifting.

SKIN TYPES

Always use skin preparations suited to your particular type of skin to get the best results. The condition of your skin will vary from time to time, especially during and after major changes in your life, such as pregnancy. You may sometimes have to change the skin creams and lotions you use to match your current skin condition. The following guidelines will help you select from the various oils and creams that I give recipes for later in this chapter.

Dry or Sensitive Skin
Dry or sensitive skin is fine, sometimes thin skin that can react to harsh soaps or other beauty products. It needs protecting to help prevent the early appearance of dry lines.

Normal Skin
Normal skin is neither dry nor oily. It is usually trouble-free, clear, and unblemished.

Oily Skin
Shiny, sallow, and prone to open pores, oily skin attracts grime and often suffers from pimples and blackheads. The bonus is that oily skin will remain youthful looking longer.

Combination Skin
"Combination skin" is the name given to facial skin with a greasy central panel, which, like oily skin, has a tendency to have pimples, blackheads, and open pores. The rest of the face can be quite dry and sensitive, especially for people with red hair, so the skin needs balancing.

Allergic Skin
Allergic skin is very delicate, fine skin that is prone to allergic reactions.

FACIAL OILS

One of the best ways to care for facial skin and to treat imbalances is a light facial massage. It has a soothing effect, but the bonus is a dramatic improvement in the skin's condition.

Use one of the oils described below, according to your skin type. Note that for each skin type, I have singled out essential oils that have proved to be especially popular and effective with my clients. These oils tie in with oils you are probably familiar with from using during your pregnancy. The other recommended oils are also suitable to try. Certain oils appear under more than one skin type because their balancing nature makes them suitable for many types of skin. The carrier oil I have recommended is jojoba—it is one I use and particularly recommend as a facial oil, but almond or apricot oil can be substituted.

Facial oil can be used at any time, but leave it on for at least one hour before putting makeup on. The most practical time to use facial oil is probably at night after cleansing the face, which also means oil can sink into restful skin.

The facial massage doesn't have to be a lengthy job or done as in a beauty salon. Just stroke the oil into the face, neck, and forehead with gentle, upward, and circular movements. Avoid the eyes. Leave the oil on the face for as long as you can or at least ten minutes (a good time to do this is while relaxing in an essential oil bath). Then blot the face with a tissue to remove the residue oil before getting into bed. If your skin is very dry, you may find that all the oil has soaked in, but blot the skin anyway—any surplus oil may find its way around the eyes during the night and can cause puffiness.

Use the facial oil two or three times a week. Choose an oil to suit your current skin condition. If you use oils to normalize an oily skin, monitor the skin's progress, and change to different oils if the skin's condition changes.

Dry or Sensitive Skin

To ½ tablespoon (10 milliliters) of jojoba oil (or almond or apricot oil), add 2 drops of either rose or sandalwood oil, or 1 drop of sandalwood oil and 1 drop of neroli oil, or 1 drop of sandalwood oil and 1 drop of rose oil. Other suitable oils are Roman chamomile, jasmine, and ylang-ylang.

Normal Skin

To ½ tablespoon (10 milliliters) of jojoba oil, add 2 drops of lavender oil, or 2 drops of geranium oil, or 1 drop of neroli oil and 1 drop of lavender oil, or 1 drop of geranium oil and 1 drop of neroli oil. Other suitable oils are sandalwood, rose, and jasmine.

Oily Skin

To ½ tablespoon (10 milliliters) of jojoba oil, add 2 drops of ylang-ylang oil, or 2 drops of geranium oil, or 1 drop of lemon oil and 1 drop of lavender oil, or 1 drop of cypress oil and 1 drop of geranium oil. Another suitable oil is sandalwood.

Combination Skin

To ½ tablespoon (10 milliliters) of jojoba oil, add 2 drops of sandalwood oil, or 2 drops of geranium oil, or 1 drop of geranium oil and 1 drop of ylang-ylang oil, or 1 drop of cypress oil and 1 drop of rose oil. Other suitable oils are lavender and neroli.

Allergic Skin

To ½ tablespoon (10 milliliters) of jojoba oil, add 1 drop of chamomile oil and 1 drop of sandalwood oil.

FACE CREAMS

It is better to use creams on the face during the day; oils are better used at night. Take note of the following points:

🌿 The essential oils singled out for each skin type are those that have proved to be especially popular and effective with my clients. The other oils recommended are also suitable to try.

🌿 When buying unperfumed creams or lotions, make sure they don't contain lanolin, which can aggravate skin rashes.

🌿 If the cream is in a plastic bottle, buy some glass jars (ask your pharmacist), because essential oils don't react well with plastic. Sterilize the jars by boiling and make sure they are dry by putting them in a low oven. Also sterilize a small, thin-stemmed plastic utensil for mixing the creams, or boil a teaspoon for five minutes to sterilize it.

🌿 When making up the oils at home, stick to a 1 percent dilution of the essential oils. For example, a 1 percent dilution of 2 ounces (50 grams) of cream would contain 12 drops of essential oil; a 1 percent dilution of 1¼ ounces (30 grams) of cream would contain 7 drops of essential oil.

🌿 Following the directions for quantities, squeeze the cream into the jar and add the essential oils. Stir very well to make sure the oil is distributed evenly and don't forget to label the jar afterward.

Dry or Sensitive Skin

To 1¼ ounces (30 grams) of cream base, add 3 drops of sandalwood oil, 3 drops of neroli oil, and 1 drop of rose oil. Other suitable oils are Roman chamomile, jasmine, or ylang-ylang.

Normal Skin

To 1¼ ounces (30 grams) of cream base, add 3 drops of neroli oil, 3 drops of sandalwood oil, and 1 drop of jasmine oil. Other suitable oils are rose, lavender, or geranium.

Oily Skin

To 1¼ ounces (30 grams) of cream base, add 3 drops of lavender oil, 3 drops of geranium oil, and 1 drop of lemon oil. Other suitable oils are sandalwood or ylang-ylang.

Combination Skin

To 1¼ ounces (30 grams) of cream base, add 3 drops of geranium oil, 3 drops of rose oil, and 1 drop of lavender oil. Other suitable oils are ylang-ylang and sandalwood.

Allergic Skin

To 1¼ ounces (30 grams) of cream base, add 2 drops of German chamomile oil and 2 drops of sandalwood oil. You may increase the number of drops to 7 if the skin tolerates the cream well. Another suitable oil is neroli.

FACIAL SCRUBS

Scrubs can be used on the face as well as on the body. If your skin looks dingy or dull, a scrub will help cleanse it by unclogging the pores and removing dirt and dead skin cells, leaving the skin fresh and glowing. The skin will then be more receptive to oils or creams.

To make a facial scrub, place 1 teaspoonful of the basic scrub mix (opposite) in a bowl. Add ½–1 teaspoonful of jojoba, almond, or apricot oil, or substitute the same amount of honey (for dry skin), yogurt (for oily skin or blemishes), aloe gel (for irritated skin), or rose water (for sensitive skin or if you need a less abrasive scrub). Add 1 drop of essential oil: rose or sandalwood (for dry skin); rose, geranium, neroli, or lavender (for normal skin); lavender, Roman chamomile, or lemon (for oily or blemish-prone skin); sandalwood, rose, or Roman chamomile (for sensitive skin); geranium or neroli (for combination skin). Mix together.

Apply the blend to the face, avoiding the area under the eyes. Leave on until the mixture feels dry (one to two minutes), then gently rub off in small circular movements with damp fingers. Don't drag or stretch the skin. If your skin is very sensitive, you may prefer to rinse off the scrub, but it won't be so effective.

Basic Scrub Mix

Mix together 4 ounces (100 grams) of oatmeal and 4 ounces (100 grams) of ground almonds. If you only have whole almonds, first remove the skins, making sure the nuts are dry or they will go bad when stored, and grind with a food processor. Store the mixture in a glass jar and keep the lid on to keep dry.

POSTPREGNANCY HAIR

The hair can be in poor condition after pregnancy. It can become lank or greasy, or it can go to the other extreme and become very dry. Some women discover that their normally curly hair becomes quite straight or vice versa. You may well notice an increase in hair loss. We all naturally lose between eighty and one hundred hairs a day, but after pregnancy you may notice even more. Don't panic. This is extremely common and a result of fluctuating hormone levels as well as possible nutritional deficiencies. Your hair will recover, but it may need a little help. Here are a few tips:

- Eat a good, well-balanced diet with plenty of protein and vitamin B. Avoid coffee and alcohol—they can deplete stores of B vitamins.

- Get a good haircut in a manageable style, preferably one that adds bounce and volume if your hair is lank.

- Gently massage your head when you wash your hair to encourage the blood supply to the scalp.

AROMAHELP

Essential oils can help restore the condition of your hair. Try the following suggestions for prewash conditioners, hair rinses, and shampoos, and tips about brushing.

Prewash Conditioners

Prewash conditioners help the hair become more manageable and shiny with a marked improvement in condition.

For dry or greasy hair and to help stimulate the scalp if there is hair loss, add 10 drops of rosemary oil and 10 drops of lavender oil to 3 tablespoons (60 milliliters) of almond oil and 2 tablespoons (40 milliliters) of jojoba oil.

For dry hair or dandruff, add 10 drops of tea tree oil and 10 drops of lavender oil to 3 tablespoons (60 milliliters) of almond oil and 2 tablespoons (40 milliliters) of jojoba oil.

Pour about 1 tablespoon (20 milliliters) of the chosen mixture into a small bowl. Using the fingertips, massage the oil gently into the scalp. Wrap the hair in a towel, and leave for at least one hour before washing the hair. Use this treatment at least twice weekly if your hair is in poor condition.

Hair Rinses

My mother used to rinse my hair in water and apple cider vinegar to keep it squeaky clean and shiny. Apple cider vinegar actually helps restore the acid mantle—the protective barrier that is removed with alkaline shampoos—and is helpful for itchy scalps or dandruff.

To 8 ounces (240 milliliters) of warm water, add 1½ tablespoons (30 milliliters) of cider vinegar. Add 2 drops of one of the following recommended essential oils: sandalwood, lavender, rosemary, geranium, or Roman chamomile (for dry or normal hair); lemon, cypress, lavender, or rosemary (for oily hair); tea tree, lavender, sandalwood, cypress, or rosemary (for a dry scalp or dandruff); tea tree, Roman chamomile, rosemary, lemon, or lavender (for thinning hair); rose or jasmine (for an indulgent treat). Use as a final rinse (that is, don't rinse it out), working it well into the hair.

Shampoo

To about ½ tablespoon (10 milliliters) of very mild baby shampoo, add 1 drop of any of the essential oils recommended for the hair rinse above (select the oil according to hair type). Stir well. Wash as usual (pouring shampoo onto the hair before adding water can make it easier to wash).

Fragrant Brushing

To help stimulate the circulation on the scalp, put 1 drop of rosemary oil onto a hairbrush. Bend your head forward, and brush the hair downward toward the floor.

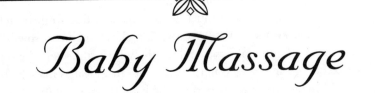

14

Baby Massage

Some of the most enjoyable times for you and your baby can come through the closeness of a cuddle at feeding time, whether you breast- or bottle-feed. Touch is very important for tiny babies, and when given and received by the parents, it helps the bonding process. Aromatherapy massage can help.

In the last few years, worldwide research has confirmed that babies who are regularly massaged eat and sleep better than those who aren't. Research has also shown that colic and constipation are reduced through massage. Yehudi Gordon, a London obstetrician, is enthusiastic about baby massage and agrees that "massage helps parents communicate with their baby, thereby strengthening the bonding process."

Early bonding is especially important for the mothers of premature babies. In 1988 a research report from the United States demonstrated the effectiveness of early infant-mother stimulation through talking, rocking, eye contact, and massage. New research from The Touch Research Institute at the University of Miami shows that massage also plays an important role in physical development, proving that it can have major health advantages. It appears that massage encourages more efficient absorption of food (massaged premature babies gained on average 47 percent more weight per day than those who did not receive massage). Massaged babies were also more responsive, active, and alert and suffered less anxiety.

BABY MASSAGE OILS

The aromatic baby massage oil (below) is perfect as a general massage oil when your baby is happy, although it will also help calm and relax her when she is not. This formula helps keep skin free from bacteria that cause diaper rash and will leave the skin clean and sweet smelling. Use it instead of mineral-based baby oils, which although they are good at keeping the baby "waterproofed" are not ideal as massage oils because they clog the pores. Try the colic baby massage oil (below) for babies with colic or other tummy troubles.

It is useful to make up a bottle in advance because having a massage oil on hand saves time. Keep it somewhere cool, with the cap tightly screwed on. Place it out of the reach of young children.

Babies and young children should always have very low amounts of essential oils. Never be tempted to use more. The amounts given in the recipes are the maximum amounts recommended for babies under one year of age. As with homeopathic remedies, less is better than more.

Aromatic Baby Massage Oil

To 5 tablespoons (100 milliliters) of almond oil, or 4 tablespoons (80 milliliters) of almond oil and 1 tablespoon (20 milliliters) of jojoba oil, add 2 drops of either Roman chamomile, rose, neroli, or lavender oil, or 1 drop of rose oil and 1 drop of Roman chamomile oil. If you prefer a smaller quantity, just use 2½ tablespoons (50 milliliters) of almond oil, or 1½ tablespoons (30 milliliters) of almond oil and 1 tablespoon (20 milliliters) of jojoba oil, and add just 1 drop of either rose, Roman chamomile, lavender, or neroli oil.

Colic Baby Massage Oil

To 5 tablespoons (100 milliliters) of almond oil, or 4 tablespoons (80 milliliters) of almond oil and 1 tablespoon (20 milliliters) of jojoba oil, add 2 drops of either tangerine, mandarin, or chamomile oil. If you prefer a smaller quantity, just use 2½ tablespoons (50 milliliters) of almond oil, or 1½ tablespoons (30 milliliters) of almond oil and 1 tablespoon (20 milliliters) of jojoba oil, and add just 1 drop of either tangerine, mandarin, or chamomile oil.

TIPS FOR MASSAGING YOUR BABY

🎕 When the time is right, give your baby a massage. Choose a time when she is content (perhaps after a bath or during a diaper-free playtime). Don't attempt to massage the child if she is tired, hungry, or fretful, although once you are both used to massaging, you may find that the baby can be comforted by it (such as a tummy or lower-back rub for colic).

🎕 Make sure you aren't tired or in a hurry, or your baby will sense your mood and the experience of massage will not be as happy as it should be.

🎕 Have everything you need ready before you begin: towel, oil, clean diaper, and clothes.

🎕 Make sure the room is warm.

🎕 You should have short nails. Remove any jewelry to avoid scratching the baby.

🎕 Don't massage for longer than ten minutes or your baby will get bored.

🎕 If your baby doesn't enjoy the massage, stop at once and try again another time.

🎕 Maintain eye contact with your baby when she is facing you. Smile or talk and let the child know that this is something to feel happy about.

🎕 The safest way to massage your baby is to sit on the floor with your legs outstretched. Place a large towel over your lap and lay the baby on top. If you find that position to be a difficult one, then try putting the baby on a large towel in the middle of the bed, but don't ever leave her alone there. Even the smallest of babies can somehow manage to wriggle to the edge.

🎕 If the phone rings in the middle of the massage, take your baby with you. Remember to wipe your hands and wrap the child in a towel; otherwise you may have an oily baby slipping right out of your arms.

- You don't need to be a practiced masseuse—just do what you think feels good to your baby. Massage gently and lovingly, and build to a gentle rhythm. Always massage upwards toward the heart.

- Most important of all, reassuringly talk or sing to your baby throughout the massage, and generally make it an enjoyable experience for both of you.

HOW TO MASSAGE YOUR BABY

You will soon find your own baby massage routine, but the following suggestions may help you in the beginning:

- Start by laying your baby on his back so that he can see what you are doing.

- Using both hands—one on either leg—start from the ankles and massage a small amount of oil upward to the tops of the legs. Then glide your hands down again to the feet. There should never be any pressure in the downward glide in either adult or baby massage, because it goes against the flow of circulation. Repeat three or four times.

- Take each foot with all of your fingers. Support the front of the foot and massage the sole in circular movements with your thumbs, first in one direction then the other. Repeat three or four times. This

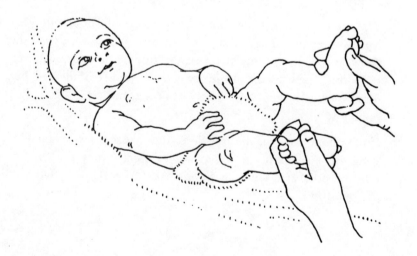

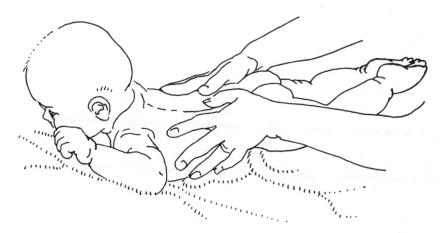

is a very calming movement for your baby and one you may find yourself returning to again and again when he needs comforting.

- Starting at the feet, stroke your hands up the legs to the abdomen, and using the palm of one hand, gently massage the abdomen in a clockwise direction. This movement is very useful when your baby has colic or is constipated.

- Move up to and circle the shoulders. Gently glide down the arms to the wrists and up to the shoulders again. Repeat three to four times.

- If your baby is still quite happy, turn him over with his head facing your feet, making sure his head isn't squashed, or lay him across your lap (obviously, in this position you can only use one hand for massage).

🌿 Massage the back of the legs from ankles to bottom. Place your hands on the top of the buttocks and glide them, with one hand on either side of the spine (unless he is lying across your lap, in which case just use one hand and keep the other free to secure him), up to the neck, out over the shoulders, and back down the sides of the body to the buttocks. Repeat.

NOTE: Don't massage the baby's hands—there is a risk that oil may be passed from hand to mouth or eyes. I also believe it's best not to massage the face because oil can get into the eyes and mouth and some babies dislike having large hands come down on their faces.

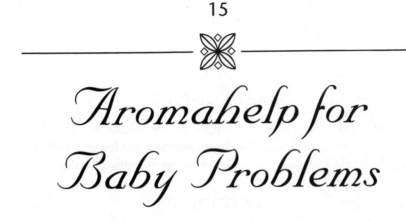

15

Aromahelp for Baby Problems

Essential oils, with their gentle calming and healing properties, can help your baby when he or she is overtired or not feeling well. They can also help keep the nursery smelling sweet and fresh. If your baby can't be comforted by the suggestions discussed in this chapter or seems to be ill, then your first call should be to the baby's doctor. Babies can become ill surprisingly fast. Don't worry about being a nuisance to the doctor—in eighteen years of being a doctor's wife, I have never heard my husband complain when an anxious mother has called him, even at three in the morning.

Seek immediate medical help if your baby or child has any of the following:

- Fever (100° Fahrenheit and above)

- Unexplained drowsiness

- Severe headaches

- Convulsions or seizures

- Altered responsiveness or irritability

- Severe vomiting or diarrhea

* Dislike of light
* Refusing feedings
* Obvious pain and distress

BABY SNIFFLES

Having a cold must be very frustrating for babies because they can't blow their noses. Some babies get the sniffles even without having a cold, and they find it difficult to breathe when they are sleeping or eating.

AROMAHELP

Use essential oils in a vaporizer in your baby's room or in the room where you feed him or her to help kill airborne bacteria, freshen the air, and help the child breathe a little easier. A vaporizer can be used and then removed before your baby goes into the room. Add 2–4 drops of either lemon, eucalyptus, lavender, or tea tree oil to a vaporizer or bowl of hot water.

BUMPS AND BRUISES

Apply an essential oil cold compress as soon as possible to reduce swelling and bruising.

AROMAHELP

Add 2–3 drops of lavender oil to 8 ounces (240 milliliters) of cold water. Agitate the water to mix the drops. Lay a cloth on top of the water to pick up the oils. Squeeze out the excess water and lay the cloth on the bruised area. Repeat as necessary. *Do not massage any swelling*.

CONSTIPATION

Persistent constipation or constipation with obvious distress and pain needs medical treatment.

In the absence of medical problems, intermittent constipation in young babies can be due to lack of fluids. Give frequent drinks of water or diluted fruit juice. Older babies and toddlers will benefit from more soluble fiber in their diet. This can be found in oatmeal, apples, bananas, and carrots. *Do not give bran.*

Toddlers can become anxious during toilet training and will "hang on," not opening their bowels for several days. This can mean passing painful movements, which in turn leads to them holding back again. Keep a relaxed attitude and let your child see that bowel function is individual and normal.

AROMAHELP

If your baby is prone to passing infrequent hard stools, encourage bowel movement with gentle massage.

Use a little of the constipation massage oil (below) and massage the lower abdomen and lower back in a clockwise direction twice a day for three to four days (see also chapter 14, "Baby Massage").

A warm bath with 1–2 drops of lavender oil diluted in 1 tablespoon (20 milliliters) of whole milk can help ease any pain. If your toddler is expressing anxiety and is frightened of opening his or her bowels, give a warm, comforting lavender bath whatever the time of day.

Constipation Massage Oil
Add 1 drop of Roman chamomile oil and 1 drop of mandarin oil to 1 tablespoon (20 milliliters) of carrier oil. Use a little of this blend twice a day.

CRADLE CAP

Cradle cap is common in newborn or small babies and is characterized by flaky patches on the scalp that come off in large pieces. The scalp is often greasy.

AROMAHELP

- Massage the scalp with the aromatic baby massage oil (see page 114), which has already been blended with an equal amount of jojoba oil. Massage about a teaspoonful into the scalp—not just the hair—very, very gently once or twice a day.

- Try using the cradle cap shampoo (below). Always shake well before using and only apply a small amount. Avoid the eyes and rinse well after shampooing. Use daily for one week or until the scalp looks clearer. Then use occasionally as the need arises.

Cradle Cap Shampoo
To 2½ tablespoons (50 milliliters) of baby shampoo, add 1–2 drops of tea tree oil and mix well.

DIAPER RASH

All babies get a sore bottom from time to time, but consult your doctor if the rash won't clear up. Here are some tips to help:

🐝 If your baby develops diaper rash, change diapers frequently. Never leave the baby in a wet diaper, especially a soiled one. Allow as much diaper-free time as possible—sore and chapped skin needs air.

🐝 Try to keep your baby's bottom as dry as possible.

🐝 If you are using cloth diapers, make sure they are well rinsed and completely free of powdered detergents or chemical cleaners.

🐝 Wipe your baby's bottom clean with cotton balls dampened with water or jojoba oil (which is particularly good). Anything dry will drag and irritate sore spots.

AROMAHELP

🐝 Use some Roman chamomile baby oil (see page 126) sparingly when changing your baby's diaper.

🐝 Apply the diaper rash cream (see page 123) to ease soreness and fight bacteria that causes diaper rash. Use the cream sparingly a couple of times a day, depending on the soreness of the bottom. To be extra safe, test the cream on a small area first—babies' skins vary and some sore bottoms should just be kept clean, dry, and well aired.

🐝 For babies over three months of age, try the diaper rash bath (see page 125). For babies over six months of age, 1 drop of tea tree oil can be substituted for the lavender or Roman chamomile oil.

🐝 If you are using cloth diapers, try soaking them in a bucket of water (having first removed any solid matter) to which you have added 6–8 drops of either lavender or tea tree oil or 3 drops of lavender oil and 3 drops of tea tree oil (this combination smells nicer). Allow the diapers to soak for two to three hours before washing them as usual. This will help disinfect the diapers. You can also add lavender oil to the final rinse after washing. If you rinse the diapers by hand, add 1–2 drops of oil to a large bowl of water. If you use a washing machine, add 4–5 drops of oil along with the fabric conditioner.

Diaper Rash Cream
To 2 ounces (50 grams) of unperfumed cream (one that doesn't contain lanolin), add 2 drops of German chamomile oil and 2 drops of lavender oil. If your health care provider thinks that the rash may be caused by a yeast infection, add 4 drops of tea tree oil instead.

Diaper Rash Bath
To 1 tablespoon (20 milliliters) of whole milk, add 1 drop of lavender oil or 1 drop of chamomile oil. Agitate well and add to a warm bath.

DIARRHEA

Severe diarrhea with or without vomiting in young babies always needs medical treatment. Babies can quickly become dehydrated and very ill.

If your child is not too unwell, a warm bath or gentle tummy massage with essential oils can be comforting and help relieve cramping pains.

AROMAHELP

Aromatic Bath
Add 1–2 drops of chamomile oil to 2 ½ tablespoons (50 milliliters) of carrier oil. Massage a little of the oil into baby's tummy. *Don't massage if your baby has recently vomited or seems to be feeling sick.*

ECZEMA

I am often asked if there are any essential oils that will ease a child's eczema. There are, but I feel it is better to take the child to a qualified aromatherapist for expert advice and to let the therapist see the condition of the skin. She or he will then make up the correct oils.

INFANTILE COLIC

Sometimes healthy babies of between six and fourteen weeks wail for long periods every night and can't be comforted. They are not thirsty, they don't appear to have gas or to feel sick, and even a clean diaper and a cuddle fail to comfort them. The crying usually occurs in the early evening and follows a set time pattern—in fact, you could almost set your watch by it. The baby may stop for brief time while being rocked, but this break is usually short lived. There is no known physical cause of these episodes, which can be very distressing, especially for a first-time mother who probably already feels insecure about her mothering skills.

In some cases, however, there may be a physical reason for this regular pattern of crying. With infantile—or three-month—colic, the baby has gas and is in pain, although it is often difficult to tell. If your baby cries regularly, assume that he or she has colic and take appropriate action.

Massage is widely used in Europe for the treatment of colic. In 1989 Danish physician Dr. Jan–Helge Larson demonstrated the success of belly massage (carried out over the clothes without oil) and whole-body massage with oil. He also determined that parents needed support and understanding while their children were suffering from colic. He established that there can be several causes of colic, ranging from insufficient burping to the parents transmitting their insecurity to the baby. At Dr. Larson's clinic, parents were shown how to massage, how to help their baby pass gas, and how to correctly position the baby for feeding.

If you have a baby who cries regularly or who may be suffering from colic, try the following suggestions:

❧ Give the baby a belly massage. There is no need to undress the child for this massage. Sit down, with plenty of room on either side of your elbows, and hold the baby in your lap, tummy downward and body sticking up a little. Massage his abdomen with one hand, starting in the middle at the navel and then gently working around in larger and larger circles in a clockwise direction. Dr. Larson recommends doing this massage fifteen to thirty minutes after a feeding.

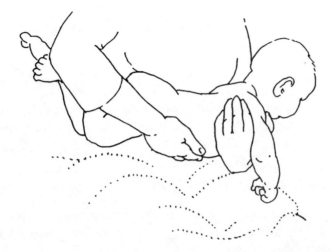

🌿 Keep calm. The baby may cry when you begin any of these remedies, but hopefully he will stop as you get them under way.

🌿 Take his diaper off. By very gently bending one or both knees up toward the tummy and making cycling movements, you can help determine whether the baby has trapped gas or is having trouble opening the bowels. Only do this movement a few times.

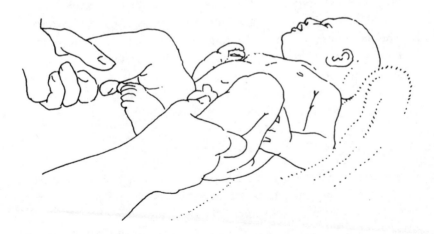

🌿 After a feeding, allow sufficient time for the baby to bring up gas before laying him down. Not even adults can burp on demand. Even if the baby doesn't bring up milk with a burp, never lay him down on his back because he could choke. Always lay him on his side.

❧ Movement can help, so try putting him in his carriage and pushing it back and forth (in the past I've done this with my foot while peeling potatoes at the kitchen sink), or park the carriage next to a switched-on dryer—the noise can be comforting.

❧ Sometimes foods that are passed through breast milk can upset a baby, particularly spicy foods such as curry and wind-producing foods such as sprouts. Check your diet to see if there is any connection with his crying.

❧ If you are bottle-feeding, ask your baby's doctor for advice.

❧ Not all babies suffer from colic. Some small babies cry because they are hungry or thirsty, so try feeding him or offering him some cooled boiled water.

❧ Don't worry about spoiling your baby by picking him up to comfort him. You can't spoil a tiny baby—he is not aware enough to manipulate you—and if he is crying, it is because he is trying to tell you that something is upsetting him. If a cuddle soothes him, don't feel guilty about giving him what he needs.

Rest assured that this awful time will end—usually, it seems, at around three months. Sometimes the only thing to do is to adapt your life around your baby's crying episodes by preparing meals before the expected crying time and planning important activities before or after them. Try not to feel that the baby is ruling you; rather; view these changes as measures of self-preservation. If you have gone back to work, don't blame yourself for these episodes. Babies still cry for hours on end when their mothers stay at home.

AROMAHELP

❧ Undress your baby and lay her on a warm towel. Massage the lower back, then turn her over and massage the abdomen in a gentle clockwise movement. These actions help dispel gas. Let the baby suckle at your breast after the massage. She may fall asleep in your arms, and you can then put her straight to bed. This massage can be done without oil or you can use the preprepared aromatic baby massage oil (see page 114) or the Roman chamomile baby oil (see page 126).

🌿 Give your baby a warm bath. For babies of three months or over, add just 1 drop of Roman chamomile oil to 1 tablespoon (20 milliliters) of milk. Agitate well; then place this mixture into the warm bathwater. Never put undiluted essential oils into a baby's bathwater. If the oil doesn't disperse properly, it could get into the baby's eyes. Also never use essential oils in a bath for a baby under three months of age.

🌿 Calm your baby down by scenting her room. Add 1–2 drops of neroli oil to a diffuser or on a cotton ball placed near a radiator. If you have other young children put the cotton ball well out of their reach.

🌿 Looking after a crying baby can be exhausting. If you become too upset or tired, ask someone in the house to look after your baby for a short time while you leave the room. Then try to relax for a few minutes. An inhalation may help calm you. On a tissue or clean handkerchief, put 1 drop of any of the following essential oils and sniff: petitgrain, geranium, mandarin, rose, bergamot, ylang-ylang, lemon, lavender, rosemary, or grapefruit.

🌿 When your baby has calmed down, run yourself a warm bath. Add 4–5 drops of any of the following oils to the water: petitgrain, geranium, mandarin, rose, bergamot, ylang-ylang, lemon, lavender, rosemary, or grapefruit.

Roman Chamomile Baby Oil
Add 2 drops of Roman chamomile oil to 5 tablespoons (100 milliliters) of almond oil. Mix well.

MINOR BURNS OR SCALDS

Seek immediate medical treatment for anything but minor burns and scalds.

AROMAHELP

Lavender's soothing properties can quickly take the sting out of burns and will help calm any distress.

Babies Under One Year Old

Add 2 drops of lavender oil to a bowl of very cold water and use a small cloth as a compress to lay over the burned area. Repeat several times. If you like, you can add a little aloe vera gel to the lavender. Do not apply this to babies' fingers—they might ingest the gel.

Babies Over One Year Old

If the burned area is accessible, hold it under cold water for as long as you can. *It is recommended that burned areas be held for at least ten minutes under cold water. Being realistic, this is sometimes impossible with a young child.* Make up a solution of 2 drops of lavender oil in a bowl of very cold water. Lay a cloth on the water and apply to the burn as a compress. If you like, smear a little aloe gel with lavender onto the burn.

Aloe Gel with Lavender

Add 2 drops of lavender to ½ tablespoon (10 milliliters) of aloe gel. This is good for minor burns and sunburn.

MINOR CUTS AND SCRATCHES

Essential oils of tea tree and lavender have antiseptic, antibiotic, and antifungal actions.

AROMAHELP

Wash and clean minor wounds with a tepid solution of 2–3 drops of lavender or tea tree essential oil diluted in 8 ounces (240 milliliters) of water.

If necessary, use a little healing gel or cover with gauze or a bandage.

Healing Gel

Add 6 drops of lavender oil and 6 drops of tea tree oil to a 2-ounce (50-gram) jar of aloe gel. Mix well. Keep the jar in a cool place ready for family first aid.

SUNBURN

If your child has severe sunburn or shows signs of being unwell, you should seek professional medical help. Babies and little children quickly become ill and dehydrated if they have too much sun.

If the sunburn is minor, cool and soothe any affected areas as quickly as possible. Keep the child cool and quiet, and give plenty of fluids. Try the following remedies:

🐝 As with other burns, a lavender essential oil compress laid on the skin can help take the redness and sting away (see compress under "Minor Burns or Scalds," above).

🐝 Apply plain aloe vera juice well diluted in water liberally to the skin.

🐝 Put the child into a tepid bath with 2 drops of lavender oil. *In this instance it is best not to dilute the oil in milk first.* Gently pat the child dry, dress in loose clothes, and keep cool. Repeat the bath after two hours if necessary.

🐝 Make up a fine spray-mist bottle containing 8 ounces (240 milliliters) of cold water and 2 drops of lavender oil. Shake the bottle very well to mix the oils. Use the mix to spray burned but unbroken skin on the back, trunk, legs, and arms. *Do not use on the face or fingers, or on very young babies.*

TEETHING

There is no set age when teething begins. Some babies are born with teeth; for others the first teeth won't emerge until they are twelve months old. In general, most babies cut their first tooth at around five or six months, when you may notice a number of symptoms. You may find that your baby becomes irritable or fretful, dribbles a lot, chews on anything he or she can get hold of but especially the fists and hands, scratches the ears, and may even develop flushed cheeks. Take care, though, not to blame other symptoms on teething. If your baby is feverish or suffers from vomiting, diarrhea, or lack of appetite, consult the child's doctor.

If your baby is teething, offer something hard to chew on: a raw carrot, a cooled teething ring, or a hard biscuit. Rubbing the gums with a cool, clean finger can also help.

AROMAHELP

🌿 Add 1–2 drops of Roman chamomile or lavender oil to a vaporizer or bowl of hot water. Place it in your baby's room.

🌿 Use the massage oil for teething (below) but only on babies six months of age or over. Rub just a smear (no more than 2 drops) along the jawline to the ear of a teething baby. Do not rub on the upper cheekbone near the eye or near the mouth.

Massage Oil for Teething

To 5 tablespoons (100 milliliters) of sweet almond oil, add 1 drop of lavender oil and 1 drop of Roman chamomile oil. Mix well.

WAKEFUL AND RESTLESS TODDLERS

Older babies and young children have difficulty settling at night for a number of reasons. They could be hungry, thirsty, frightened of the dark, or frightened that you may not return, or it could simply be that life downstairs sounds too exciting to miss. Some children become hyperactive at bedtime and all efforts to keep them in their beds fail.

If your child is clearly not tired, allow him or her to join the family for a while, to work out extra energy. There is little comfort in forcing a miserable child to stay in bed. However, a bedtime routine can be quite comforting for children, even very young ones, so try not to make a habit of allowing a restless child to break bedtime routines.

Children and babies seem to instinctively know when their parents are going out. They have difficulty settling when they sense it, so try not to hurry bedtime on these occasions. Get them ready for bed well before you leave the house.

AROMAHELP

Most children unwind with a warm bath. I don't recommend using essential oils in the bath for babies under three months of age, but after that the oils can be very helpful. Use discretion, however, with small babies who become distressed every night. They cry for very different reasons than toddlers cry; regular aromatherapy baths are not recommended for them.

Mothers who are having trouble getting their children to sleep may give them a Roman chamomile bath (below) every other night for a week, then for two or three nights the following week. At the end of two weeks, the child should be back into a regular sleep pattern. Roman chamomile oil, though very mild and suitable for children, is best when used as needed. A child should not be given a chamomile bath as a matter of course.

Calming Bath

To a cup or bowl containing ½–1 tablespoon (10–20 milliliters) of whole milk, add 1–2 drops of Roman chamomile oil. Stir well and add to the warm bathwater. Then mix well in the water.

A WORD OF CAUTION

Some people use essential oils on a baby's bedding and clothing. I don't recommend this practice because undiluted oils might come in contact with the baby's skin. When using cotton balls perfumed with essential oils to scent a baby's room, never put them directly into the baby's bed and take care with the amount of essential oil used (whether you use cotton balls or a vaporizer). For babies of under one year, use only 1–2 drops and no more. For babies over one year, increase the amount to 3–4 drops.

16

A Reference Guide to Essential Oils

There are many essential oils available on the market, but in this chapter I have only listed the oils that are mentioned throughout the book. These are the oils that I have successfully used on my clients and can personally recommend.

A–Z OF ESSENTIAL OILS

Some, but not all, of the properties and general uses of essential oils are discussed below. Remember that unless you are very familiar with essential oils, it is best, especially during pregnancy and for young children, to only use them as directed in the recipes and instructions for baths, oils, creams, and gels given in this book.

BENZOIN (STYRAX BENZOIN)

Part of plant used: Gum resin exuded from the trunk of the benzoin tree

Where produced: Thailand, Malaysia, East Indies

Aroma: Warm, vanilla smell

Price: Middle

Main properties and effects: Antiseptic, diuretic, expectorant, healing, sedative

Main uses: Benzoin is a pulmonary antiseptic and can be used as an inhalation to help expel mucus and relieve respiratory congestion. When used in a postpartum massage, it creates a feeling of warmth and comfort for those who feel emotionally cold. It is helpful for those with poor circulation and stiff, cold joints. It helps heal dry, cracked skin and sores, and it blends well with lemon oil in a cream for rough, cracked hands. Use postpartum in a cream or gel for cracked and sore nipples. Benzoin is thick and will be slow to pour from the bottle. It will solidify when kept under cold conditions but will thin readily when brought to room temperature. It keeps well.

Ways to use: Inhalations, body massage, skin care

Preconceptual care: No

Pregnancy: No

Labor: No

Postpartum care: Yes

Babies: No

BERGAMOT *(CITRUS BERGAMIA)*

Part of plant used: Expressed from the rind of the fruit

Where produced: Southern Italy, northern and western Africa

Aroma: Fresh, citrus, sweet smelling

Price: Middle

Main properties and effects: Analgesic, antiseptic, antidepressant, antispasmodic, antiviral, deodorant, healing, refreshing, uplifting

Main uses: Bergamot is the oil used to scent and flavor Earl Grey tea. It is very uplifting for those who feel depressed or physically or mentally fatigued. It is indicated for some types of eczema and for skin conditions that have been brought on by stress. Use well diluted, alone or with lavender, to help infected pimples, boils, and wounds. It is one of the best oils to help relieve urinary and genital infections, particularly for those prone to frequent attacks of cystitis. Used as a bath oil during feverish illness (colds, flu, and such) bergamot is cooling. It makes an ideal bath oil to help ward off depression during convalescence.

Ways to use: Body massage, facial oil, skin care, vaporization, baths, showers, local application, compresses

Preconceptual care: No

Pregnancy: Yes (as a room freshener and, sparingly, for cystitis)

Labor: No

Postpartum care: Yes

Babies: No

CAUTION: Bergamot must not be used before sunbathing or using a tanning bed because it can cause uneven pigmentation.

CHAMOMILE, ROMAN *(ANTHEMIS NOBILIS);* GERMAN *(MATRICARIA CHAMOMILLA)*

Part of plant used: Distilled from the dried flowers

Where produced: Italy

Aroma: Pungent dried grass/herbal smell

Price: Middle to expensive

Main properties and effects: Antiseptic, analgesic, anti-inflammatory, antispasmodic

Main uses: Like lavender, chamomile oil is a first-aid kit in a bottle. Its aroma is either liked or loathed. It contains an anti-inflammatory substance called azulene, which gives it its familiar blue color. Roman chamomile can, however, vary from pale watery blue to colorless. German chamomile has a thicker consistency and contains a higher proportion of azulene. It should be a deep blue, but it tends to turn a greenish yellow-brown as it ages or after frequent exposure to the air. German chamomile also tends to be expensive. Do not confuse Roman and German chamomiles with chamomile maroc, which is not from the same family (always check to make sure your suppliers' lists give the Latin names of essential oils). Chamomile's anti-inflammatory action helps calm, soothe, and control many skin problems and allergies. Its pain-relieving actions help soothe dull, nagging pain from muscular aches, toothaches, teething pain, headaches, chronic orthopedic problems, and so forth. Its antispasmodic action is excellent for period pains, indigestion, flatulence, and especially infantile colic. Chamomile is a gentle sedative for young or old. It relaxes those who are stressed, anxious, irritable, or having trouble sleeping. It can help calm overtired or fretful children before bed.

Ways to use: Body massage, facial oil, skin care, baths, showers, local application, compresses, vaporization

Preconceptual care: No

Pregnancy: Yes

Labor: No

Postpartum care: Yes

Babies: Yes

CLARY SAGE *(SALVIA SCLAREA)*

Part of plant used: Distilled from the whole plant

Where produced: Europe

Aroma: Sweet, nutty, exotic, heavy

Price: Middle

Main properties and effects: Antiseptic, antidepressant, antispasmodic, emmenagogue, aphrodisiac, uterine tonic

Main uses: Clary sage is used in aromatherapy in preference to common sage, which is very strong and can be toxic even in small doses. Clary sage is nontoxic but should still be used in small quantities— a 1 percent dilution is ideal. If used in too high a quantity it can be euphoric, leaving one feeling lightheaded. It should not be used in treatment before driving a car or before drinking alcohol. Although suitable for both sexes, I think of clary sage as a feminine oil. It helps regulate hormonal imbalance (it contains natural plant hormones resembling estrogen). It is helpful for premenstrual tension and is strongly indicated for menopausal symptoms. It can help lower high blood pressure. Its antidepressant action makes it one of the best oils to use for postpartum blues. During labor it can be used as a compress to help relieve pain. Reputedly an aphrodisiac, its aroma is sensual and its relaxing, antidepressant, and euphoric actions do seem to help dispel tension a couple may be experiencing.

Ways to use: Body massage, facial oil, baths, showers, vaporization, compresses

Preconceptual care: Yes

Pregnancy: No

Labor: Yes

Postpartum care: Yes

Babies: No

CYPRESS *(CUPRESSUS SEMPERVIRENS)*

Part of plant used: Distilled from the needles, cones, and twigs of the tree

Where produced: Europe

Aroma: Woody, spicy, medicinal

Price: Middle

Main properties and effects: Antiseptic, antispasmodic, astringent, deodorant, diuretic

Main uses: Cypress is used for problems associated with a sluggish, poor circulation, such as fluid retention, cramps, thread veins, varicose veins, and ulcers. Its locally constricting action on capillaries makes it invaluable for treating hemorrhoids. Its powerful astringent action is similar to that of witch hazel. Used postpartum it helps heal sore perineal areas. Its properties can help control excessive amounts of body fluid, such as in menorrhagia (heavy periods). It suits oily and combination skin. As a bath oil it has a deodorant effect, helps to reduce perspiration, and is relaxing and refreshing. It has a gentle sedative action on nervous tension. Its antispasmodic action will help relieve coughing.

Ways to use: Body massage, skin care, local application, compresses, baths, showers, vaporization

Preconceptual care: No

Pregnancy: Yes (after five months)

Labor: No

Postpartum care: Yes

Babies: No

EUCALYPTUS *(EUCALYPTUS GLOBULUS)*

Part of plant used: Leaves and twigs of the tree

Where produced: Although native to Australia, the tree now grows in places, such as North Africa, the Mediterranean, and California

Aroma: Strong distinctive smell, probably known to most people because it is widely used in pharmaceutical products to help clear a stuffy nose

Price: Inexpensive

Main properties and effects: Antiseptic, antibiotic, analgesic, anti-inflammatory, antiviral, diuretic, stimulating

Main uses: Eucalyptus is primarily used for its effect on the respiratory tract, to help clear mucus and ease congestion. Correctly diluted, it is suitable for all ages. This oil is very strong, so always use on the skin in a 1 percent dilution or less. It can be used as an antiseptic wash for cuts and scrapes, and when well diluted in water, gel, or cream, it can be applied (with bergamot) to cold sores or pimples, particularly if they are inflamed. Added to a massage blend with other oils, its warming and anti-inflammatory action helps ease stiff joints (especially in rheumatism) and aching muscles. Eucalyptus is cooling to the body, so it is helpful during feverish illnesses. Use in a very low dilution in baths for urinary infections, particularly when they are accompanied by a fever. It can be used either in the bath or as a cool compress to help take the unpleasant itch out of chicken pox blisters (please consult your aromatherapist for advice about quantities to suit the age of your child). Used in room sprays or vaporizers, it will help cleanse the air and cut down on airborne bacteria. Ideal for places where germs lurk—bathrooms, doctors' waiting rooms, offices, schools, and so on. Mix in equal parts with bergamot and lemon for a more agreeable aroma.

Ways to use: Body massage, local washes, vaporization, compresses, skin care, baths (very low dilution)

Preconceptual care: No

Pregnancy: Yes

Labor: No

Postpartum care: No

Babies: Yes

GERANIUM (PELARGONIUM GRAVEOLENS)

Part of plant used: Distilled from the whole plant

Where produced: Grown in several places, the best coming from Réunion Island

Aroma: Fresh, flowery

Price: Middle

Main properties and effects: Antiseptic, antidepressant, astringent, diuretic, fortifying, healing, refreshing, toning, uplifting

Main uses: Geranium is probably one of the most useful oils in aromatherapy; it is helpful for many ailments. Its effect on the body is to balance. Postpartum and in general treatments for everyone, its uplifting aroma can cheer and relieve depression and fatigue, whether used in a massage bath or vaporizer. It stimulates the lymphatic system, relieves fluid retention, and relieves congestion in engorged breasts. It is frequently used in cellulite treatments. It has a regulating action on hormonal balance and is often used alone or in a blend to relieve premenstrual and menopausal symptoms. It is excellent for all types of skin. Used in facial oils, lotions, and creams, its action helps balance the production of sebum (natural oil) in the skin. Blended into a carrier oil and used after a bath or shower, it leaves a delightful fragrance on the skin. Used in compresses, local washes, and creams, it can help heal wounds and sores. Geranium can be stimulating so it is best avoided in a massage toward the end of the day. Conversely, it makes a good reviving bath oil to use before going out for the evening. Its scent is liked by most people. It blends well with most oils but is quite powerful and will tend to dominate other oils, so use in moderation if you are using it in a blend. It makes a good oil to spray around the house to freshen up rooms, particularly in old houses, and is useful as an insect repellent.

Ways to use: Face and body massage, facial oil, skin care, baths, showers, local application, compresses, vaporization

Preconceptual care: Yes

Pregnancy: Yes (in low dilution for freshening rooms and after six months for local applications)

Labor: Yes

Postpartum care: Yes

Babies: No

JASMINE *(JASMINUM OFFICINALE)*

Part of plant used: Flowers

Where produced: Egypt, Morocco, India

Aroma: Highly fragrant and sweet

Price: Very expensive

Main properties and effects: Antidepressant, antiseptic, antispasmodic, aphrodisiac, helpful during labor, increases breast milk flow, general tonic

Main uses: With its heavenly fragrance, jasmine is much loved by the perfume industry. For something so delicate, jasmine oil is very strong—only a few drops are needed either when used alone or in a blend. It has an uplifting, calming, and boosting effect on the emotions and makes an ideal choice to add to a postpartum massage blend because it also helps increase breast milk flow. During labor it will help boost confidence, relieve pain, and help expel the placenta. Its effects are beneficial for painful periods and helpful for the emotional symptoms sometimes experienced during menopause. Reputedly an aphrodisiac, its use is strongly indicated in preconceptual care or for emotionally related sexual problems. Added to a cream or used in a facial massage oil, jasmine is very good for dry and sensitive skin.

Ways to use: Body and face massage, baths, showers, vaporization, skin care

Preconceptual care: Yes

Pregnancy: No

Labor: Yes

Postpartum care: Yes

Babies: No

LAVENDER (*LAVANDULA OFFICINALIS*)

Part of plant used: Distilled from the flower heads

Where produced: All over Europe

Aroma: Fresh and floral

Price: Inexpensive

Main properties and effects: Antiseptic, antibiotic, analgesic, antidepressant, diuretic, antiviral, antifungal, antispasmodic, healing, sedating, toning

Main uses: This gentle essential oil must rate as the one most used by aromatherapists. Lavender enhances the effects of other oils it is blended with and mixes well with the majority of oils. It has a wide range of properties, but its main effect on the body is to normalize it. Its antiseptic and healing properties help with cuts, wounds, dermatitis, eczema, diaper rash, pimples, and burns. As with tea tree oil, undiluted lavender may be used in tiny quantities directly on the skin. One of the most important oils in skin care, it helps to encourage cell renewal and minimize scars. Use in a facial oil for any skin type. Lavender will help regulate menstruation if the body is out of balance. It is used to treat all muscular aches and pains, particularly acute pain. It is recommended for use in labor. It makes a physically and mentally relaxing bath oil for anyone. It can help relieve fluid retention and ease aching legs and feet. Use in a massage or compress to relieve headaches and migraine. Its gentle but effective sedative action encourages restful sleep in the young and elderly. It will help calm and relieve the pain of infantile colic. Use to treat yeast infections and athlete's foot in local washes, creams, and gels.

Ways to use: Body and face massage, local washes, baths, showers, vaporization, skin care

Preconceptual care: No

Pregnancy: Yes

Labor: Yes

Postpartum care: Yes

Babies: Yes

LEMON *(CITRUS LIMONUM)*

Part of plant used: Expressed from the rind

Where produced: Mainly in the Mediterranean

Aroma: Fresh and citrus

Price: Inexpensive

Main properties and effects: Antiseptic, antibacterial, antifungal, astringent, diuretic, stimulant, tonic

Main uses: Although the lemon fruit has a sharp acid taste, the oil is known to cut down acidity in the body and is very refreshing. Used widely in beauty care, it is astringent and healing and is reputedly an age retardant. Add it to face creams and masks to whiten and soften dull skin (used in neck creams especially). It makes an excellent addition to hand creams. When added to a mild skin tonic, such as orange flower water, lemon oil will reduce oiliness, freshen greasy skin, and tone open pores. Use after shampooing to rinse greasy hair. Because of its mild bleaching action, lemon oil is a longtime favorite in hair rinses for fair hair. When added to a bath or massage blend, lemon oil's toning and invigorating action can stimulate a sluggish circulation and help reduce fluid retention and cellulite. Keep a lotion containing lemon, geranium, and cypress oil in the refrigerator to help soothe throbbing varicose veins. Lemon in a vaporizer or room spray can cut down on airborne bacteria and freshen the atmosphere. Its fresh aroma can ease the nausea experienced in morning sickness. A 2 percent dilution in water can be used to bathe cuts and scrapes (if the wound is infected, use previously boiled and cooled water). Using the same 2 percent dilution, soak a cotton ball and hold it across the bridge of the nose to help control nosebleeds (pinch the nostrils together to help constrict the capillaries). Seek medical advice if a nosebleed is severe or if nosebleeds happen frequently. Undiluted lemon oil can be used to help remove warts and verrucas but not moles (see your doctor). Put 1 drop onto the wart with a cotton ball or the corner of a tissue, or add it to a gauze pad or bandage before applying. Avoid the surrounding healthy skin and keep the wart (or verruca) covered. This is best done twice a day, but if you are rushed in the morning, do it faithfully every evening for successful results. The wart will eventually drop off. It is difficult to forecast how long this will take, but the average time is a month.

Ways to use: Body massage, skin care, baths, showers, local application, vaporization

Preconceptual care: No

Pregnancy: Yes

Labor: No

Postpartum care: Yes

Babies: No

MANDARIN *(CITRUS NOBILIS)*

Part of plant used: Expressed from the rind

Where produced: Mostly the United States and South America

Aroma: Citrus, fresh, mild

Price: Inexpensive

Main properties and effects: Antiseptic, refreshing, tonic, digestive stimulant, mild relaxant

Main uses: Tangerine *(Citrus reticulata)* has the same therapeutic properties as mandarin. Both mandarin oil and tangerine oil are very gentle and can be used in massages for both young and old. They are useful for all kinds of stomach upsets (whether caused by food poisoning or emotional upsets) and constipation. During pregnancy and postpartum, these two oils make refreshing, calming, and fortifying baths. They are the first choice of ingredients in creams and oils to help keep body skin supple during pregnancy. Mix with geranium oil for a delicious-smelling body oil or lotion. Their very gentle diuretic effects make them suitable additions to massage blends and baths to help disperse minor fluid retention. When used in a vaporizer, their aroma is pleasant and cheering.

Ways to use: Baths, body massage, showers, skin care, vaporization

Preconceptual care: No

Pregnancy: Yes

Labor: Yes

Postpartum care: Yes

Babies: Yes

MARJORAM, SWEET *(ORIGANUM MAJORANA)*

Part of plant used: Flowering tops and leaves

Where produced: Europe, the Mediterranean

Aroma: Sweet, warm, powerful

Price: Middle

Main properties and effects: Analgesic, antiseptic, antispasmodic, strong sedative, menstrual stimulant, vasodilator

Main uses: Do not confuse sweet marjoram with Spanish marjoram *(Thymus mastichina),* which, although called marjoram, is from the much stronger thyme family. Sweet marjoram is a strong oil to be used sparingly. It is warm, comforting, and calming and encourages sleep, so it is as helpful to the insomniac as it is to those who suffer from anxiety, stress, and unhappiness, whether deep-rooted or acute. Its properties can help reduce high blood pressure, headaches, and migraines. It relieves nagging muscular aches (particularly cramps), arthritic pain, and sporting injuries. Use mixed in a blend with chamomile or lavender, but never massage acute injuries or inflamed joints until the swelling has subsided. Instead use on a compress to ease swelling and pain. When gently massaged on the lower abdomen, its soothing action can help constipation, colic (adults), and menstrual pain. Described as dulling to sexual desire, it might not be the best oil to massage your lover with, unless he or she is suffering from stress, insomnia, or torn knee ligaments.

Ways to use: Body massage, baths, showers, compresses, vaporization

Preconceptual care: No

Pregnancy: No

Labor: No (although some birth units use marjoram during early labor)

Postpartum care: Yes

Babies: No

NEROLI *(CITRUS AURANTIUM)*

Part of plant used: Distilled from the flowers of the bitter orange tree (orange flower water is produced from the distillation water)

Where produced: Mainly Italy and Tunisia

Aroma: Warm, floral

Price: Very expensive

Main properties and effects: Antiseptic, antidepressant, antispasmodic, anti-inflammatory, aphrodisiac, relaxing, calming

Main uses: Neroli is used by the perfume and cosmetic industry (one of the classic oils used in eaux-de-cologne). With its beautiful aroma and the pleasing sensations it arouses, I call this the "antianxiety oil." It rates among the best oils for dispelling fear, shock, nervous tension, depression, and panic attacks, and will calm and relieve the unwelcome effects that these stresses bring to the body, such as labored breathing, insomnia, mental fatigue, irritability, and stomach upsets. Its value in therapy as a face and body oil is enormous. Neroli helps stimulate healthy new skin cells and is widely used by aromatherapists in skin care creams. A facial massage with this luxurious oil not only treats the skin but relaxes the mind, body, and soul at the same time. Diluted to 1 percent, it can be used on very delicate skin and soothes inflamed areas.

Ways to use: Body and face massage, baths, showers, skin care, vaporization

Preconceptual care: Yes

Pregnancy: Yes

Labor: Yes

Postpartum care: Yes

Babies: Yes

PETITGRAIN *(CITRUS AURANTIUM)*

Part of plant used: Leaves and twigs of the same bitter orange tree that gives us neroli oil

Where produced: Italy, Tunisia

Aroma: Floral, fresh, mild

Price: Inexpensive

Main properties and effects: Antiseptic, antidepressant, sedative, deodorant, refreshing, tonic

Main uses: Because petitgrain oil comes from the same tree as neroli, it is not surprising that it shares the same properties but to a lesser degree. It is not as sedating or calming and its perfume is lighter and fresher than neroli's. It leaves one feeling both relaxed and invigorated, making it a good choice for someone who wants a massage with the aroma of neroli but who doesn't necessarily need its more powerful therapeutic and calming effects. As a bath oil, it has deodorant and refreshing properties and is liked by both men and women. A rather big plus to using petitgrain is that it is so much cheaper than neroli, which means that it is more accessible to most people. It makes a refreshing additive to facial oils, creams, and aftershave lotions, particularly for greasy or pimply skin.

Ways to use: Body and face massage, baths, showers, vaporization, skin care

Preconceptual care: No

Pregnancy: Yes

Labor: No

Postpartum care: Yes

Babies: No

ROSE *(ROSA DAMASCENA)*

Part of plant used: Distilled from the flower petals

Where produced: Bulgaria, North Africa, Morocco, France, Turkey

Aroma: Very fragrant, floral

Price: Very expensive

Main properties and effects: Antiseptic, antibiotic, antidepressant, anti-inflammatory, aphrodisiac, menstrual stimulant, tonic

Main uses: *Rosa damascena* is therapeutically the best rose oil; *Rosa centifolia* is highly fragrant but therapeutically inferior. Rose is a beautiful and much-loved flower with a feminine fragrance to match. Rose oil is chosen by my patients purely for its scent. It is a powerful antidepressant, especially useful where there is grief, sadness, shyness, and uncertainty. Its feminine qualities make it useful for all premenstrual, menstrual, and menopausal problems. Men are not excluded from benefiting from this wonderful oil—it is said to increase sperm production. It is postpartum uplifting, and I can think of no nicer present for a new mother than a bunch of roses and an aromatherapy product containing a good rose oil (avoid synthetic rose oil—it smells cheap, is cheap, and can give you a headache). Rose is highly antiseptic and, although its high price precludes its use as an everyday antiseptic, it comes into its own in a cream for sore, inflamed skin. As a skin tonic, it is suitable even for babies and makes a wonderfully fragrant additive to a plain moisturizing cream. Use for dry, sensitive skin that is prone to thread veins. Rose is tonic to the digestive system, especially the liver. It is especially useful for ongoing digestive complaints that result from long-term stress. For a deliciously relaxing and indulgent bath, add 3–4 drops to the water. Rose water is collected at the same distillation as rose oil and makes a refreshing and mild skin tonic, particularly suitable for dry and sensitive skin. It is also good for red, inflamed eyes: Apply to cotton balls, place over closed eyes, and relax for ten minutes.

Ways to use: Face and body massage, skin care, vaporization, baths

Preconceptual care: Yes

Pregnancy: No

Labor: Yes

Postpartum care: Yes

Babies: Yes

ROSEMARY (ROSMARINUS OFFICINALIS)

Part of plant used: Distilled from flower heads and leaves

Where produced: France, Spain

Aroma: Strong, clean, herbal

Price: Inexpensive

Main properties and effects: Antiseptic, analgesic, general stimulant, menstrual stimulant, astringent, diuretic, tonic

Main uses: An invigorating and stimulating oil, rosemary helps get things moving. As a result of its effect on circulation, it is widely used in treatments for fluid retention and cellulite. It helps relieve the congestion around varicose veins. It makes an invigorating massage for those who lack muscular tone or who feel sluggish in mind as well as in body. Its nonsedating, pain-relieving qualities help soothe sports injuries, especially because its diuretic action helps disperse the fluid that collects around the injury site. Its properties help general aches, pains, and stiffness, whether brought on by physical activities or the result of joint and rheumatic conditions. As a general tonic, it helps banish feelings of fatigue and is helpful during convalescence. Combined with geranium, it makes a good reviving bath or shower early in the morning or after work. It makes a good postpartum bath oil but because it is stimulating, do not use it at the end of the day or the oil's effects may keep you awake. Rosemary is legendary for its ability to help stimulate the memory and allow for clear thought. In massages and compresses, it can help relieve headaches and migraines and clear a stuffy head. As a hair tonic, rosemary can help treat dandruff and encourage hair growth. Just as chamomile is traditionally used in hair rinses for blond hair, so rosemary is used for dark hair.

Ways to use: Body massage, inhalation, vaporization, compresses, baths, showers

Preconceptual care: No

Pregnancy: No

Labor: No

Postpartum care: Yes

Babies: No

SANDALWOOD *(SANTALUM ALBUM)*

Part of plant used: Wood chippings from the tree

Where produced: East India

Aroma: Warm, exotic, woody

Price: Middle

Main properties and effects: Antiseptic, anti-inflammatory, antidepressant, aphrodisiac, antispasmodic, sedating

Main uses: For thousands of years, sandalwood has been used in traditional Indian medicine and religious ceremonies. It is a very healing and soothing oil, both mentally and physically. It is a strong urinary and pulmonary antiseptic and has the ability to clear the body of mucus. It can soothe and treat dry coughs, catarrh, and sore throats, and it can ease urinary tract infections. During pregnancy and postpartum, use in a warm bath or a lower-abdominal massage to help cystitis. It has a calming action on the digestive system and can help flatulence, diarrhea, heartburn, colic, and nausea. With its anti-inflammatory actions, sandalwood is particularly suited to dry, inflamed, or allergic skin, but because of its antiseptic and astringent properties, it is also helpful for acne and oily patches. It makes an excellent facial oil blended with jojoba, and if you like its rather pronounced smell, it makes a nourishing additive to a moisturizing cream. As an antidepressant and relaxant, sandalwood is an oil to choose when stressful problems have led to a lack of direction or emotional and sexual dullness.

Ways to use: Facial and body massage, skin care, baths, showers, vaporization

Preconceptual care: Yes

Pregnancy: Yes

Labor: No

Postpartum care: No

Babies: No

TEA TREE *(MELALEUCA ALTERNIFOLIA)*

Part of plant used: Distilled from the leaves of the tree

Where produced: Australia

Aroma: Strong, medicinal

Price: Inexpensive

Main properties and effects: Antibiotic, antiseptic, antifungal, antiviral, disinfectant

Main uses: The highly antiseptic powers of tea tree oil have been known to the Australian Aborigines for thousands of years. It would appear to be a panacea for many infections. Research has shown it to be more powerful than many household disinfectants and antiseptics. It can be used to treat skin and scalp infections, septic cuts, boils, and wounds as well as warts and verrucas. Australian dermatologists have proved it to be more effective at controlling acne than many other skin preparations. As an antifungal agent, it proves to be highly successful at treating conditions such as yeast infections and athlete's foot. It may be used undiluted in tiny amounts on scrapes, minor burns, pimples, and small wounds (be careful with sensitive skin). It can encourage a quick recovery from viruses and bacterial infections because it appears to be able to boost the body's immune system.

Ways to use: Baths, body massage, local washes, inhalations, vaporization, compresses, skin care

Preconceptual care: No

Pregnancy: Yes

Labor: No

Postpartum care: No

Babies: Yes

YLANG-YLANG *(CANANGA ODORATA)*

Part of plant used: Distilled from flowers from the tree

Where produced: Java, Madagascar

Aroma: Sweet, strong, fragrant

Price: Inexpensive to middle

Main properties and effects: Antiseptic, antidepressant, aphrodisiac, lowers blood pressure, sedative

Main uses: Ylang-ylang is used on its own or in blends to help calm acute or long-term physical symptoms that arise from anxiety, nervous tension, fear, shock, anger, and emotional problems. It helps normalize a racing heartbeat and rapid breathing experienced when one is frightened and under stress. It helps to lower blood pressure. Its antidepressant, relaxant, and aphrodisiac properties work well together, particularly on someone who is overworked, tired, and under stress. Its exotic perfume adds a lingering fragrance to body lotions, creams, and bath oils. Added to facial oils and creams, it is balancing and can be used for all skin types. I find it ideally suited to oily and combination skins.

Ways to use: Face and body massage, baths, and showers, skin care

Preconceptual care: Yes

Pregnancy: Yes

Labor: Yes

Postpartum care: Yes

Babies: No

USING PERCENTAGES WHEN MAKING OILS AND CREAMS

It is advisable to use a very low concentration of essential oil when making up massage oils, creams, and lotions for use during pregnancy. Baths and footbaths are not so critical, because a set number of drops is usually used in a large volume of water. Dilutions can be formulated by using percentages to adapt to the size of the bottles or containers you have at home.

PERCENTAGES FOR NONPREGNANT WOMEN (OVER SIXTEEN)

Most aromatherapy massage oils for nonpregnant women are made to a 2½ percent concentration (that is, 2½ percent of the total volume of massage oil should be made up of essential oils). Determine how much your container holds. Fill it with a carrier oil, then add half the number of drops of essential oil as there are milliliters of carrier oil. For example:

🌺 To a 3½-ounce (100-milliliter) bottle of carrier oil, add 50 drops of essential oil.

🌺 To a 1½-ounce (50-milliliter) bottle of carrier oil, add 25 drops of essential oil.

🌺 To a ⅓-ounce (10-milliliter) bottle of carrier oil, add 5 drops of essential oil.

PERCENTAGES FOR PREGNANT WOMEN

During pregnancy and the postpartum period—and for those with sensitive skin—I suggest you use massage oils with a 1 percent concentration of essential oil. Adding approximately half the number of drops of essential oil that you did for the 2½ percent concentration above will give the correct proportions. For example:

❧ To a 3½-ounce (100-milliliter) bottle of carrier oil, add 25 drops of essential oil.

❧ To a 1½-ounce (50-milliliter) bottle of carrier oil, add 12 drops of essential oil.

❧ To a ⅓-ounce (10-milliliter) bottle of carrier oil, add 2 drops of essential oil.

Glossary of Medical Terms

Analgesic: Pain relieving

Antibiotic: Kills pathogenic bacteria

Antidepressant: Mood elevator

Antifungal: Stops growth of mold or fungi

Anti-inflammatory: Reducing or preventing inflammation

Antiseptic: Wound cleaning; prevents microbe development

Antispasmodic: Relieves smooth-muscle spasm

Anti-viral: Destroys certain viruses

Aphrodisiac: Substance that stimulates sexual desire

Astringent: Contracts blood vessels and body tissue

Bactericide: Substance that inhibits growth of bacteria

Balancing: Maintaining or returning to a state of equilibrium

Decongestant: Substance that reduces congestion

Diuretic: Substance that aids production of urine

Emmenagogue: Substance that induces menstruation

Engorged: Congested

Expectorant: Substance that encourages coughing up of mucus

Sedative: Substance that lessens excitement or functional activity

Resource Guide

ALLISON ENGLAND
AROMATHERAPY PRODUCTS

I can supply all essential oils mentioned in this book, plus carrier oils and glass bottles. I also have a full range of ready-prepared creams, massage oils, and gels to treat a wide variety of complaints, including a full range of skin-care creams. These are available by mail order from:

Allison England Aromatherapy,
The Trees,
97 Main Street,
Little Downham, Ely,
Cambridgeshire CB6 2SX
Telephone and fax: 01353 699236
E-mail: AllisonEngland@dial.pipex.com.
Web site: www.allison.england.dial.pipex.com

Please write or phone for a current price list.

Allison England Retail Products
Pure essential oils
Pure essential oil synergie mixes
Massage and body oils
Aromatic gels
Bath products

Hypo-allergenic skin care
Gift packs

Special Products for Pregnancy, Labor, New Mothers and Babies
Anti-Stretch Mark Gel/Cream
Anti-Stretch Mark Oil
Pregnancy Relaxing Bath Oil
Labour Day Massage Oil
After-Delivery Healing Bath Drops
Aroma Baby Products
Pregnancy Bath/Shower Gel
Chamomile and Rose Baby Oil
Chamomile and Rose Baby Bath

U. S. SUPPLIERS OF ESSENTIAL OILS

Aroma Vera
5901 Rodeo Road
Los Angeles, CA 90016
Telephone: (800) 669-9514
(310) 280-0407
Fax: (310) 280-0395
Web site: www.aromavera.com

Original Swiss Aromatics
P. O. Box 6842
San Rafael, CA 94903
Telephone: (415) 459-3998

Santa Fe Fragrance, Inc.
P. O. Box 282
Santa Fe, NM 87504
Telephone: (505) 473-1717

Tiferet International
210 Crest Drive
Eugene, OR 94705
Telephone: (503) 344-7019

AROMATHERAPY ASSOCIATIONS, COURSES, SEMINARS, AND CLASSES

To find an aromatherapist in your area who is qualified in pregnancy massage, contact:

The American Society for Phytotherapy and
Aromatherapy International, Inc.
P. O. Box 3679
South Pasadena, CA 91031

Aromatherapy Seminars
3379 South Robertson Boulevard
Los Angeles, CA 90034
Telephone: (800) 677-2368

Pacific Institute of Aromatherapy
P. O. Box 6723
San Rafael, CA 94903
Telephone: (415) 459-3998
Web site: www.pacificinstituteofaromatherapy.com

OTHER ORGANIZATIONS

Academy of Certified Birth Educators
2001 East Prairie Circle, Suite 1
Olathe, KS 66062
Telephone: (800) 444-8223
Web site: www.acbe.com

The Academy of Certified Birth Educators offers courses on childbirth education.

Global Maternal/Child Health Association, Inc.
P. O. Box 1400
Wilsonville, OR 97070
Telephone: (503) 682-3600
Web site: www.waterbirth.org

Devoted to protecting the well-being of women and children, the Global Maternal/Child Health Association (GMCHA) provides computer referrals to midwives, doctors, and birth centers in the United States and abroad; rents and sells portable tubs for labor and birth; and offers courses and workshops on water birth for both professionals and parents.

International Cesarean Awareness Network
1304 Kingsdale Avenue
Redondo Beach, CA 90278
Telephone: (310) 542-6400
E-mail: ICANinfo@aol.com

The International Cesarean Awareness Network (ICAN), formerly the Cesarean Prevention Movement, offers information about and support for cesarean prevention and vaginal births after cesarean sections through their newsletter, conferences, and training for childbirth educators.

La Leche League International
14 N. Meacham Road
Schaumburg, IL 60173
Telephone: (312) 455-7730
Hotline: (800) LA LECHE
Web site: www.lalecheleague.org

La Leche League International (LLLI) offers support for women who want to breast-feed or who are having problems with breast-feeding. Call the hotline between 9:00 A.M. and 3:00 P.M. (CST) for breast-feeding help or a referral to a local La Leche support group. LLLI also publishes many informative books on breast-feeding.

Midwives Alliance of North America
P. O. Box 175
Newton, KS 67114
Telephone: (888) 923-6262

The Midwives Alliance of North America (MANA) supports practicing midwives, provides information about midwifery to consumers, and offers referrals from its membership list.

Recommended Reading

For those who wish to read more about aromatherapy, massage, or food-combining diets mentioned in the text, the following books may be helpful:

Arcier, Micheline. *Aromatherapy*. London: Harnlyn, 1990.

Maxwell-Hudson, Clare. *The Complete Book of Massage*. London: Dorling Kindersley, 1989.

Stead, Christine. *The Power of Holistic Aromatherapy*. Poole, England: Javelin Books, 1986.

Van Straten, Michael, and Barbara Griggs. *Superfoods*. London: Dorling Kindersley, 1990.

Valnet, Jean. *The Practice of Aromatherapy*. Edited by Robert Tisserand. Rochester, Vt.: Healing Arts Press, 1982.

Index

petitgrain, 33–34, 144
  as antidepressant, 34, 88, 90, 144
  as deodorant, 144
  for labor, 83
  for skin care, 100, 144
  for stress, 127
pheromones, 14–15
pneumonia, 14
postpartum depression. *See* antidepressants
postpartum fitness, 96–97
  and cellulite, 97, 101–4
  and diet, 97–98
  and exercise, 98–99
postpartum pain, 24, 27, 86
pregnancy. *See also* individual conditions
    and oils
  baths during, 26
  best oils for, 32–34, 53
  and essential oils, 3–5
  limited use oils for, 34–38
  oils to avoid, 7, 39–41
productivity, 15

rose, 46, 47, 145
  as antidepressant, 15, 75, 90, 145
  as aphrodisiac, 19, 46
  for baby massage, 114
  for eyes, 145
  for hair, 112
  for labor, 75, 82
  for menstrual problems, 46, 145
  for skin care, 9, 100, 101, 108–11, 145
  for semen production, 47, 145
  for sore nipples, 95
  for stress, 15, 127, 145
rosemary, 40, 41, 146
  as antidepressant, 90
  for cellulite, 104, 146
  for fatigue, 146
  for fluid retention, 146
  for hair, 112, 146
  for memory, 146
  for skin care, 101
  for stress, 127
  for varicose veins, 146

sandalwood, 35, 47, 147
  for acne, 147
  as antidepressant, 47, 147
  for colic, 147
  for cough, 147
  for cystitis, 35, 59, 147
  for hair, 112
  for impotence, 47
  for indigestion, 63, 147

  for skin care, 35, 67, 100, 101,
    108–11, 147
  for stress, 147
semen production, increasing, 47, 145
sinuses, 65. *See also* nosebleeds
  eucalyptus for, 65, 137
  inhalations for, 28–29
  lavender for, 65
  tea tree for, 65
sitz baths, 27, 59, 61
skin care. *See also* facial massage
  almond for, 100, 111
  benzoin for, 101, 133
  body creams, 99–100
  chamomile for, 101, 108–11, 134
  clary sage for, 101
  "cold cream," 19
  cypress, 101, 108
  exfoliating, 20, 100–101
  geranium for, 100, 101, 108–11, 138
  grapefruit for, 101
  jasmine for, 100, 101, 108, 109, 139
  jojoba for, 9, 67
  lavender for, 67, 100, 101, 108–11, 140
  lemon for, 101, 108–11, 133, 140
  mandarin for, 100
  marjoram for, 101
  neroli for, 33, 67, 100, 101, 108–11,
    143
  oatmeal for, 100, 111
  olive oil for, 19, 38
  orange flower for, 67
  petitgrain for, 100, 144
  rose for, 9, 100, 101, 108–11, 145
  rosemary for, 101
  sandalwood for, 35, 67, 100, 101,
    108–11, 147
  tangerine for, 142
  ylang-ylang for, 100, 101
skin, exfoliating, 100–101
  and dry skin brushing, 102–4
  and facial scrubs, 110–11
skin, postpartum, 105–6. *See also* skin,
    exfoliating
  and facial creams, 109–10
  and facial massage, 107–9
  and facial scrubs, 110–11
  skin types, 9, 67, 106–10
stress
  bergamot for, 127
  chamomile for, 134
  cypress for, 136
  geranium for, 47, 127
  grapefruit for, 127
  jasmine for, 15